The Energy Source

Health Screen Check List

These exercises have been carefully planned and are safe and effective

However if you answer yes to any of the following questions, then you should check with your doctor before partcipating in the exercises.

Have you ever suffered from heart disease, high blood pressure, or any other cardiovascular problems?
Have you ever been troubled with any unaccountable chest pains, especially if associated with minimal effort?

Are you prone to severe headaches or fainting?

Are you pregnant or have you had a baby in the last six months?

Do you suffer from pain or limited movement in any joints?

Have you any medical condition which you think may affect your ability to exercise?

If the answer to these questions is no then enjoy the exercises.

The Energy Source

Simple daily exercise
for mind and body vitality

Clare West

Prion

First published in Great Britain in 1997 by PRION BOOKS
32-34 Gordon House Road London NW5 1LP

Copyright © Prion Books Limited 1997

Text copyright © Clare West

Illustrations by Charlotte van der Geest

Cover design by Bob Eames

A CIP catalogue record for this book is available from the British Library.

ISBN 1 85375 235 5

Printed and bound in Great Britain

CONTENTS

INTRODUCTION

Have you tried to stick to an exercise programme before and failed to keep it up? If so, can you remember what your reasons were for starting? Perhaps you felt you were overweight, or that your body was out of proportion, or too small or too weak?

Many of us embark on a fitness programme from a negative starting point. It may be that we are unhappy with our bodies, feeling that they fail to conform to some idealized image that society considers to be 'normal'. We may also believe that we are fundamentally lazy when left to our own devices and that we need bullying into shape – the old 'no pain, no gain' maxim. So we place ourselves in the hands of experts and subject ourselves to rigid exercise programmes that are often monotonous and, frequently, insulting to our intellect – programmes that separate the body from the mind, as if the body were a thing apart that we were capable of divorcing and of servicing independently from the mind. Such programmes usually require a large time commitment and may often involve the use of equipment.

Certainly, if we become very dedicated, we can briefly reach a peak of physicality on this regime, perhaps even attain this idealized 'norm'. Yet, because of our negative starting point, and the lack of an integrated approach that involves our whole being, our bodies ultimately rebel. We then spend much of our time falling short of the physical goal we set ourselves and chastising ourselves for failing. With this approach, the programme soon becomes a punishing regime that is hard to sustain.

There is, however, an alternative way of approaching fitness, one that starts out from a more supportive and positive perspective. You could begin exercising simply because you would like a stronger, healthier, more flexible body that enabled you to function to the best of your ability in your everyday life, with increased energy and vitality.

Each of us is different and the notion that there is some 'normal' physique to which we can all aspire is, quite simply, false. The body is not a fixed object but a constantly changing organism that adapts to whatever we subject it to; to the stresses it must absorb; to the diet it must process; to our individual physical weaknesses; to our age, our emotional state and our hormones – the list is endless. When left to its own devices, it is not lazy or stupid but an incredibly intelligent, self-regulating organism. The body has its own wisdom and knows what is best for it. It makes thousands of biological decisions concerning our wellbeing, every minute of the day, without our supervision. What we need to do is to become sensitive to its requirements and to support and follow them.

Because the body is in a constant state of flux, the way to maintain a level of fitness and balance is to listen to it daily and respond to its messages. By exercising a little every day you can achieve a greater awareness of your body and its needs. If you listen to it and give it regular attention, messages that might otherwise go unheard can be acted upon, and fatigue, injury or illness can be anticipated and may be avoided. With a little encouragement, your body will begin to flourish. Exercise approached from the point of view of pleasure and even

joy will be much more effective than some punishing regime. Then your body will be free to radiate energy and vitality.

This is the principle upon which the ideas in this book are based. Here you'll find a gentle and manageable way of exercising that will enable you to be fit for life. The aim is to work with your body rather than against it and to involve your whole being and sensibilities in the process. Being kind and encouraging with your body is the key to obtaining the best results. The maxim of The Energy Source is 'less is more'. A little exercise, done well and often, with focus and the right intention and with the attention of your whole being is ultimately more effective than a lot of exercise carried out at speed and without understanding. The Energy Source exercises will develop your ability to listen to your body and to respond to it. Each body is unique and you are the person most qualified to know what is good for yours.

The ideas and exercises described in this book came about after 26 years of putting my body through punishing training as a classical dancer and neglecting to support myself physically or mentally as a working professional later. I recall one day during my training, when I laughed as I released myself from an excruciating exercise and was told: 'You'll never be a dancer if you laugh.' The seeds of my rebellion were sown.

This level of physical exertion, negativity and lack of self-support could not continue for long, and by the age of 28 I had numerous injuries and was in such poor health generally that I found myself no longer able to dance. Initially, I was very despondent and resentful, but as I looked for solutions to my problem I began to see the 'gift' that my years of ballet and contemporary dance training had given me. I had an incredible wealth of knowledge of movement and experience of my own body. Armed with this knowledge, I discovered I could adapt certain dance movements so that they would work gently on any condition.

I began to listen to my body and its needs. It had taken such a dramatic low for me to begin to be kind to myself and to work my body gently, but I found that my body responded rapidly to kindness and healed itself naturally when I allowed it to do its work. I also noted that, because of the beauty and rhythm of the dance movements, I was able to sustain my own interest and attention, something I was never able to do with conventional exercise. This is how my gentle system of exercising, which eventually became known as The Energy Source, evolved.

As I read and explored other approaches to movement and exercise, I discovered that the ideas and philosophy that had developed quite naturally in me were completely in keeping with the Eastern philosophy of movement and energy and similar to those ideas used in T'ai-chi, Jan Jong, Aikido and Yoga. I developed the Energy Source ideas further during my work as a choreographer and director, where I encourage opera singers to develop their bodies and their physical skills. I always work gently and supportively with them to allow them to give their best. Now, we use the Energy Source exercises as a daily preparation for rehearsals and performances. The performers tell me that, to them, the Energy Source work is more than just a preparation for a performance, it is a preparation for life.

The Energy Source exercises in this book fall into three distinct areas – the Energy Fountain preparatory exercises featured in Chapter 1, the Daily Energy Exercises in Chapter 2, and the remedial exercises in Chapter 3.

The Energy Fountain preparatory exercises encourage the development of sensitivity to the body and an awareness of the Universal Energy around us. They provide unusual ideas and images which will help you to 'open' your body and allow the energy to flow through and revitalize you. These energy images are fundamental to the Energy Source method and are applied to the Daily Energy Exercises to increase their effectiveness. So start by familiarizing yourself with the preparatory exercises before you move on to the Daily Energy Exercises.

The Daily Energy Exercises are based on dance movements which I have modified to be gentle yet effective and are designed to promote flexibility, strength and coordination to create a supple toned body with healthy, malleable muscles. In combination with the images of the Energy Fountain, these exercises stretch and work the pressure points in the body, releasing tensions and toxins and creating energy and vitality. They work with the mind and body as one, using the powerful tool of the imagination to transform the body and tap into an endless source of Universal Energy that replenishes vitality.

In the remedial exercises in Chapter 3, the ideas of the Energy Fountain are applied to common stress-related problems. There are breathing exercises to promote deep relaxation and techniques for identifying and releasing energy blocks and stiffness or for removing a tension headache.

The first and most difficult commitment in this programme is to dedicate a small amount of time to yourself each day – about 20–30 minutes. This is harder than it sounds, as you have to consider your fitness a priority and yourself worthy of the attention. Initially, there will always seem to be more important things to do. Try to find a time of day that you know will be easiest for you, a time when you can concentrate without fear of interruptions, and then mentally reserve the time for yourself as a treat, in the way that you might take time out for a well-earned soak in a hot bath.

Remember, please don't look upon these exercises as some form of punishment and undertake them simply because you feel you really ought to be doing something about your body. If you start out this way, exercising will soon become yet another chore to try and squeeze in to an already full schedule. Then you'll start to chastise yourself for being lazy and feel guilty for failing to achieve your goal. No, my Energy Source method requires you to be gentle and compassionate with yourself.

If you still think the idea of exercise feels like self-punishment, try taking five minutes each day to sit quietly alone. Just focus on your steady breathing and try to quieten your mind. Let that be your 'treat'

at first. Do this each day until the idea of stretching and exercising during that time starts to feel pleasurable.

Be thankful initially for every moment that you do manage to dedicate to yourself. However little exercise you do, it will be one hundred per cent more beneficial than doing nothing at all! On those days when you don't manage to exercise, don't chastise yourself. Just be aware of how you feel and how you function that day without the exercise. Pick up again the next day or as soon as you can. When you recommence the exercises, take time to listen to any new stiffness or energy blocks that your body may have acquired, especially if you have been under stress. Once you have established a regular routine, it will become second nature to exercise daily and, in fact, it will feel strange if you don't, like being unable to take a shower.

Over the last nine years since I retired from dancing I have maintained my body with around 20 minutes of Daily Energy Exercises a day. This might vary from anything between 10 and 45 minutes on occasions, depending on my work schedule. However, with the old, negative 'no pain no gain' approach, a serious workout would need to involve more effort than this. A two-hour workout in the gym might leave you feeling marvellous, with all your tensions spent, but you could manage this probably only once, or at most twice, a week if you were really dedicated.

With the 'little but often' approach of the Energy Source you will find it remarkably easy to exercise for three or more hours a week and to feel invigorated and balanced every day. Like the fable of the tortoise and the hare, it may seem gentle and slow, but it is sustainable and, ultimately, it's a winning pace.

It will take a while for you to get used to the exercises, though, so don't be disappointed if you feel you have not achieved much in your first few sessions. These ideas and exercises will serve you for life, so it's worth taking your time over them. As they become familiar to you, you will gradually be able to cover more ground in your daily session. Just work in a focused way and take the opportunity to listen to your body.

Here's what some of the performers who use the Energy Source exercises have said:

It's an uplifting and revitalizing experience. I arrive at rehearsals feeling tense, hunched and small, but with these stretching and breathing exercises I expand in both body and mind. Clare gives me the opportunity to focus on and care about every part of my body and to observe my darting thoughts. I learn to direct my energy with my mind and to control and expand my breathing. After 30 minutes I feel as if I have ten times more energy than before. I am then able to learn more quickly, concentrate for longer and enjoy my work more.

Sarah Leonard, opera singer

I found the energy work made me feel simultaneously calm and exhilarated. I felt better able to concentrate, and the whole of me felt alive, ready, able, prepared. Since being introduced to the exercises I have found myself less tired at the end of a day and also noticed a greater clarity to my thoughts. It is fantastic.

Rebecca de Pont Davies, opera singer

At 60 I have tried them all – Clare's method of exercise is unique in my experience. It heightens awareness of your mental and physical condition, allowing greater personal control of your fitness. It is the only exercise programme I have enjoyed and looked forward to in its entirety.

Eve Jenkins, Costa Blanca Energy Source Group

The Energy Source exercises have been used by performers from the Covent Garden Royal Opera, English National Opera, Opera de Paris Bastille, Lontano Contemporary Music Ensemble and have been presented at The Healing Art of Opera Symposium at the Covent Garden Festival. They are also practised by the Costa Blanca Energy Source Group, Javea, Spain.

Clare West February 1997

CHAPTER 1

THE ENERGY FOUNTAIN

Only be still a moment

Before any conscious movement begins in the body, there is first a thought and an intention to move. The quality of our initial thought totally influences the way in which we will approach the movement or task. For instance, if we think that the activity is going to be hard work or difficult for us to perform, or worse, that we are not capable of doing it at all, then we will tend to contract our muscles, tensing up and blocking the flow of our energy. Our thoughts dictate the quality of energy that we put into a movement and so determine the success or failure of that task.

We may actually be giving our bodies unhelpful signals and images each time we undertake a specific task. Repeated frequently, these negative thoughts and the resulting tensions are quickly embodied by us and begin to feel normal. As a result, many of us use a lot more effort and muscle power than is actually necessary for a particular action. At some point we perceived the task to be difficult and so we now hold ourselves in a state of tension.

Tension requires large amounts of energy to sustain it – it is a kind of energy 'black hole'. As you are sitting reading this chapter, is there is a part of your body that is unnecessarily tense – the jaw, the hands, the shoulders, the stomach? This extra muscular effort and tension is clearly unnecessary in order for you to read this chapter. Tension blocks the clear flow of energy through our system and hinders the flushing-through of waste and toxins. As well as eating up energy, tense muscles produce a lot of waste products. If the outward flow of energy from that area is blocked, the muscles hold on to these toxins causing further solidifying.

In a healthy body, toxins are removed via the lymph system. This system has no muscular action of its own, but relies on free muscle action, encouraged by movement and exercise, for its drainage. Tensely held muscles gradually lose their elasticity over the years and become fibrous, hindering the work of the lymph system. A combination of tension, fibrous muscle and lack of exercise, therefore, means a less efficient disposal of toxins, which will make the body sluggish and, over time, can lead to illness – the body is literally poisoning itself. To undo the habits of a lifetime requires patience; first we must develop a sensitivity and an awareness of our bodies and how we are using them.

The most powerful tool that we have to assist in this undoing is our imagination – what I call our Mind's Eye. The images that we conjure for ourselves while we are working or exercising impact our energy, strength and wellbeing. Try this simple exercise: conjure up in your Mind's Eye an image of strength and effort. It's very likely that what you 'see' is a contracted or clenched movement; a gripped fist for strength and a furrowed brow for effort. This is an image of strength and effort to which we are frequently exposed and may adopt ourselves. There are other ways to imagine strength, though. For instance, in Eastern philosophies of movement, images of strength involve a relaxed, fluid body that uses the outward flow of energy and the natural momentum of the body's

weight. The mind is open and clear yet intent on the outward flow of energy. In this state the body is ready to deal with any eventuality.

Imagine for a moment that the energy in your body is flowing water and your body is simply a water channel. The water is flowing from an endless source and passing through you on its way to another destination. Like a river, it flows constantly away from the source, always water and yet constantly changing its nature. It can be agile and mercurial, gentle or forceful and strong. If the channel itself is weak, silted up and has fissures and flaws, the flow of water will be blocked and the current ineffective. However, if the channel is clear and strong, then the water can flow unhindered. If we develop our bodies and strengthen this channel, we can learn to harness the water's power and to move with it.

Now go back to the previous image of strength and effort – the contracted movement or gripped fist. Try to feel the difference in the energy of these two opposing images. Can you feel that the energy in the contracted image is bound and limited, rather than free-flowing? The focus of the contracted movement is inwards on itself, blocking the free flow. There is no clear channel for the energy to course through. It must churn round and round within its closed channel. It boils away with no release and the body is soon depleted. Contracted movements block the flow of energy. They are rigid and incapable of responding to any eventuality. Constricted energy is soon exhausted.

Try this simple exercise with a partner.

Stand upright, with your feet slightly apart. Make a strong fist. Hold the fist vertical, with the thumb uppermost. Hold your arm out in front of you, just below shoulder height. Straighten your arm but do not lock the elbow. Ask your partner to attempt to bend your arm, i.e. to push your fist to your shoulder, bending your arm at the elbow. Your partner should grip your wrist or forearm with one hand and start pushing from there. Resist as hard as you can, using a lot of effort. After a couple of tries your partner will succeed.

Now extend your arm out in front of you again exactly as before, keeping the arm at the same level and the fist vertical. This time, open your hand and consciously relax your arm. The hand and arm should feel energized but without tension. Again, do not lock your elbow. The important thing is that you engage your imagination and focus all your attention on the following images.

Imagine that your shoulder and arm are some sort of channel and that there is water pouring over and through your shoulder, cascading down your arm and directed out through your fingers. Send the water out way beyond yourself and see it continuing into the distance. Focus your Mind's Eye on the direction of the water's constant flow, through you and beyond. Ask your partner to repeat the test and try to force your open hand up to your shoulder by pushing from the wrist or forearm as before. Do not resist your partner by using muscle force and effort; simply focus on the direction of the flow. Your arm should feel powerful and relaxed. If your arm goes rigid, stop, shake

out your arm and try to conjure up the image and all the sensations again. If you are doing this correctly, your partner will not be able to move your arm.

Should your partner succeed in moving your arm, try again – you probably shifted your attention from the outward flow of the water on to what your partner was doing and the faces he or she was pulling in the exertion. Once you manage to focus your imagination on the outward flowing water, your fluid energy will always be more powerful and more effective than your partner's contracted efforts. Just imagine how strong we could be if we applied this gentle image to all our day-to-day activities. All the exercises in this book use this flowing water principle. The 'water' is often simply referred to as energy in the exercises. If you prefer, you could imagine some other form of energy such as brilliant light, although the fluid quality of the water energy is the most useful image with movement and exercise. This image keeps the body open and relaxed and, at the same time, it has cleansing properties to rid the body of toxins. By engaging the tremendous power of the imagination in our exercise and activities, we can transform our bodies. We can create vital, flexible and balanced bodies that serve us well.

The whole universe is made up of movement and energy. Energy is all around us, an endless source. By using the Energy Fountain preparatory exercises that follow, we can begin to become sensitive to this energy, particularly to the energy field that immediately surrounds our bodies. The exercises will develop our ability to listen to our bodies, to release tensions and restrictions and to 'open' our bodies so that they can receive a greater energy flow. By learning to access the endless source of Universal Energy, we can reclaim the vitality that is rightfully ours.

ACCESSING THE ENDLESS SOURCE OF ENERGY

The following Energy Fountain preparatory exercises will help you develop your sensitivity to the energy and awareness of your body. The exercises allow you to 'listen in' to your body and respond to its messages, while the images help you to deeply relax your muscles and still your mind. Relaxation and stillness are essential for increased vitality and energy.

The sensations you will experience in these preparatory exercises will be new to you. It will take time and practice to become familiar with them and experience their full possibilities. As you practise these exercises you will be developing your kinesthetic memory – this is the body's ability to remember a sensation and a physical movement pattern so that in the future it can reproduce it immediately without conscious thought. A simple example is learning to swim. Once the patterns are mastered, the body immediately understands all the complicated movements and sensations it must reproduce when we give it the instruction 'swim'. The same will happen with the Energy Fountain exercises. With practice,

you will be able to conjure up detailed images and sensations without difficulty. These sensations and images are used constantly to enhance the effectiveness of the Daily Energy Exercises in Chapter 2.

Work with the Energy Fountain preparatory exercises as often as you can at first to develop your awareness of your body. Ideally, practise them once a week initially until you become accustomed to them. Later you should do them about once a month to refresh your memory. Each time you return to them, you will be aware of more details and more layers than you were the previous time. It will ultimately take about 20–30 minutes to perform all of them. Choose one or two of them that you particularly enjoy as preparation for the Daily Energy Exercises or to relax and revitalize you at any time.

Try to choose a quiet room for this work, somewhere where you are unlikely to be interrupted or disturbed for at least half an hour. These exercises demand a focused concentration, which is hard to sustain at first. If you find your mind wandering away from the exercise, don't be discouraged or get angry with yourself. Simply bring your focus back, think of the images again and continue with the exercise. At first you may have to do this as much as once a minute, but your ability to focus will improve with practice.

If you are very preoccupied with other thoughts, then this is not a good time to do the preparatory work. Although the exercises can be used to release worrying thoughts and tensions, this must be your intention from the beginning. If the worries are particularly stubborn, try the Throwing Your Worries exercise in Chapter 3. If you have a tension headache or your body is feeling stiff or tense, you could begin by doing the Unblocking Energy exercise, also in Chapter 3.

When I'm exercising I always keep a notebook to hand in case I find myself distracted by other matters and losing concentration. Then if my brain interrupts an exercise to report on some practical task that I have forgotten to do, I note it down immediately and tell myself: 'I'll do it in half an hour but for now I'm concentrating.' Then I let the thought go completely. Try to see it float away from you, until it is very small, somewhere at the edge of your awareness and know that you will return to it later after you have finished.

You may find that you yawn a lot as you do these exercises. This is the body's way of getting rid of toxins as effectively as possible. Really enjoy big wide yawns and don't try to stifle them.

THE ENERGY FOUNTAIN PREPARATORY EXERCISES

The Energy Field

* Stand upright with your feet as wide apart as your hips and arms relaxed by your sides.
* Take a moment to focus on your breathing. Just allow your breath to rise and fall naturally. While you are breathing, imagine for a moment that your body does not stop at the tips of your fingers or the surface of your skin, but that it extends out from its visible surface in all directions – upwards, backwards and down into the ground. If you were able to see this area physically, it would appear as an oval, radiating out from you about two or four feet (60–120cm) – the distance is personal to you. Just take a moment to stand and breathe in a relaxed way, imagining that your breath is filling this space around you. You may feel as if you are expanding and growing as you do this. Be aware of your skin's surface and imagine it softening to allow you to breathe through its pores into this expanded area.

* When you can begin to sense this oval around you, try slowly raising one arm and imagine that this area or energy field opens and follows the movement, surrounding the arm.
* Try to imagine your slow movement causing waves through the energy field surrounding you, like ripples on a lake that extend out from you and continue after your initial movement has appeared to finish.
* Now begin to walk around slowly and take with you in your Mind's Eye the image of this energy field. Keep breathing into it, concentrating and being aware of the waves that your movements make. When you feel you have concentrated enough, come to stillness.

The Support

The feet form a very important energy connection between us and the earth. They support us and carry our body weight all day and yet they are often a very neglected part of the body.

* Stand with your feet as wide apart as your hips and arms relaxed by your sides.
* You are going to stretch the feet. Place your weight onto your left foot. Lift the right toes off the floor and stretch them forwards, away from the heel. Imagine they are elastic or chewing gum. Slowly place the elongated toes back on the floor. Now lift the heel of the same foot, leaving the toes in place. Stretch the heel backwards, away from you, and imagine you are lengthening the foot. Slowly place the heel back on the floor and take all the weight of the body onto that foot.
* Repeat the stretch with the left foot.
* Now, as you stand, be aware of the whole surface area of your feet in contact with the floor. Let your feet relax and melt into the floor. Imagine them spreading out like roots or creeping ivy, in all directions across the floor.
* Feel the pressure of your weight spread evenly through them. To check this, rock your weight backwards slightly onto the heels, lifting your toes, and then rock your weight forwards slightly onto the toes so that you are able to lift your heels. Now rock back to the centre until you are sure that your weight is centred over your feet. Be aware of the contact and pressure of the floor and of the floor supporting your weight.

* Now, try to imagine that there is an actual physical warmth coming from the floor as it supports you. Imagine, if you can, that the support of the floor is like two hands that are holding or cupping your feet. The warmth is coming through the hands into you.

Standing Light

* Stand with your feet as wide apart as your hips and arms relaxed by your sides.
* Take your Mind's Eye into the sensations in your feet. We are going to travel with the Mind's Eye through the body.
* First to the ankles. Let the ankle bones simply rest on top of the feet. Release any gripping you are aware of, particularly in the tendon in the front of the ankle. Release the calf muscle. Unlock the knees. Let the knees simply rest on top of the shin, without using any muscle tension to hold them in place. Release the front thigh muscles and release any 'holding' in the hips. Let your hips simply be placed on top of your legs and not held tense. You may find that the hips tilt forwards a little as you release them. Keep your breathing deep and confident.
* With one 'out' breath, release the stomach. Take your Mind's Eye to the base of your spine. Slowly work your way up the spine, vertebra by vertebra. Imagine the vertebrae as building blocks placed one on top of another. They are just floating there with no muscle tension involved. By now it should feel a little as if you are suspended in water. You are standing upright with no

effort or tension. You will not fall.

* With one good 'out' breath, let the shoulders fall away from the neck. Let the head rest on top of the spine, and release the muscles in the front of the neck and throat. Keep breathing confidently.

* Finally, on an 'out' breath release the jaw... Breathe... Release the eyeballs... Breathe... Release the forehead and scalp... Breathe... Release the tongue. Keep your breathing alive and, without gripping your muscles, go into the next exercise in this relaxed state.

The Energy Fountain

* Take your Mind's Eye way down into the earth beneath your feet, as deep down as you can. Imagine that you can see something brilliant and shining far below you such as a light source or sparkling, shimmering water. See this light source clearly.

* As you breathe in, consciously draw the light source through the earth towards the soles of your feet. As it comes closer, imagine you can see very clearly the quality of the crystal water or shimmering light. Now use the 'in' breath to draw it into your body through the centre of the soles of both feet. The light source is warm and invigorating. It travels up inside your legs, buoyant, lifting your ankles up out of your feet and lifting your knee joints out of your shins. It travels up through your thighs, fills your hips and lifts them up out of your legs. The force of the water is strong and supports your limbs. As it courses up your spine, your vertebrae are enlivened and lifted. As it circles through the chest it creates space.

It circles within your neck and the back of your head, lengthening them. It creates space as it fills your head and face. The water is so powerful and wonderful that some of it escapes out through the crown of your head directly upwards and onwards into the universe. It is a constant force, lifting and supporting you. The water passes through you as if you were a clear water channel and clears debris on its way. It is a fountain of energy.

* Some of the water cascades downwards towards the earth. Feel it stroke your face and pour off your shoulders. It courses down your arms and chest, softening them. It drops from your fingertips back into the earth, to its source. This is an endless fountain, an endless circle. Stay with the image for a few moments longer, trying to be aware of all the sensations of the Energy Fountain simultaneously.

* To come out of this exercise, gradually let the image of the water recede down through your body. Let it drain back into the earth and come to stillness. Take a moment to breathe before moving on to the next exercise.

The Star

* Return to the image of the light source way beneath you in the earth. As you breathe in, draw the light towards you. This time, you decide what energy it is. Is it light, water, electricity, a laser?

* Using the 'in' breath draw the energy up through the soles of your feet then up through your body, following the same upward path as before.

* Now, using a very firm 'out' breath, send the energy out in five directions, through the following five points:

Up the back of your neck and out through the top of your head (1).

Up through the centre of your body and out down both arms (2 and 3). Guide it out of your body through your fingertips.

Back out through the soles of both feet (4 and 5) and into the earth.

* On an 'in' breath draw the energy in through the feet. Then breathe out firmly and again imagine sending the energy out through the five points simultaneously. Do this several times until you can feel the energy moving out in all five directions at once. See in your Mind's Eye the energy travelling out beyond you into the universe. Feel your body growing and elongating with each 'out' breath, rather than collapsing as the lungs empty.

* Now, as you breathe in and out, begin slowly to raise your arms on each 'out' breath. Imagine, if you can, that the force of the energy travelling through you has increased and that it is raising your arms for you.

* When your arms reach the horizontal position, level with your shoulders, you will be forming a five-pointed star, sending energy out in all directions. I call this position Open Star Standing. Stay and just breathe in this position for a moment. Try to sense the quality of the energy and feel all the directions simultaneously. Draw the energy in until it fills your body with the 'in' breath, then send it out through the five points firmly on the 'out' breath.

* If you feel able to continue, move on to The Shooting Star exercise. If not come out of this exercise slowly as follows:

Coming out of The Star

As The Star is a very invigorating exercise, the increased oxygen and energy may make you feel a little dizzy at first, so it's important to come out of it slowly.

* To release it, imagine that the force of the energy is gradually turned down. Continue breathing and, with each breath, allow the ebb and flow of energy to diminish. Allow your arms to lower slowly as the flow of energy becomes more gentle. Keep breathing. Take your time. When your arms reach the sides of your body, fingertips pointing downwards, allow the energy to recede into the earth, to its source. Breathe calmly and normally for a moment before you start to move around.

The Shooting Star

* To continue the The Star sequence, as you stand in the Open Star position, feeling the energy flowing through you and out in all five directions, imagine that the flow of energy is turned up again even stronger. As the force becomes more powerful, let it slowly raise your arms. Continue to send energy out through the arms on each 'out' breath and allow the energy to lift your arms until they are both pointing straight up towards the sky. Eventually you will feel the energy moving through you in a direct line: through the top of your head and through your fingertips into the sky, and also through the soles of your feet down into the earth. Feel that you are a clear channel for the energy, directing it through you and out into the universe.

* Hold this position and breathe for about a minute, trying to be aware of the sensations and of energy flowing in both direction. When you feel you have had enough, come out of this slowly as described above.

The Energy Fountain and The Star are very powerful ways of sensing energy moving through the body. These images are referred to constantly in the Daily Energy Exercises as the basis for understanding the flow of energy. They can also be used on their own, at any time of day. If you do them in a five-minute break during the day, you will feel refreshed and invigorated. Try thinking of The Energy Fountain while you are walking down the street or standing in a queue. It will certainly make you feel light on your feet.

Wave Breathing

This is a relaxing breathing exercise that involves the whole body and a good one to finish with after any exercise session.

* Stand with your feet parallel and as wide apart as your hips, arms by your sides.
* As you breathe in, let your knees bend as deeply as they can, without raising your heels off the ground. At the same time, allow your arms gently to rise in front of you. Imagine your arms are resting on top of water so that they feel buoyant and supported from underneath without effort.

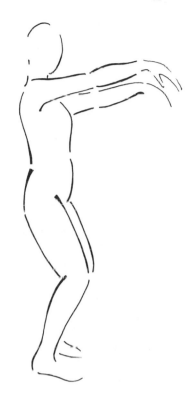

* As you breathe out, press the heel and palm of each hand down through the 'water' and, at the same time, straighten your legs. Feel a slight resistance as you lower the arms, as if pushing them against the water's surface.

* Continue the movements described above with each breath. Try to to find a natural rhythm that combines the breathing with the movement so that your arms and hands are an expression of the movement of the breath. Focus on the wave-like nature of the movement. There is no top or bottom to the wave, only continuous motion, and the breath is relaxed and easy, not forced. The turn-around moment of the wave – the ebb into the flow – is almost imperceptible. Allow the breath to move in the same way

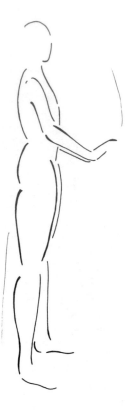

so that it is not held at the top or at the bottom, but a continuous wave.

* When you feel you have focused enough for today, come to stillness at the end of an 'out' breath. Stand still for a moment and take the opportunity to thank your body for its service to you.

You are ready to face the world.

Chapter 2

THE DAILY ENERGY PROGRAMME

The Energy Fountain preparatory exercises in Chapter 1 develop our ability to sense the Universal Energy that is all around us. This energy is constantly there for us to draw on. It courses continually through the body en route to other destinations so that the body acts as a channel for this energy. Once we begin to become aware of this energy, we also become aware of the need to develop our bodies so that we can utilize this energy. To harness the energy to the full, we need to maintain a clear, strong, sensitive body or channel, and this is the aim of the Daily Energy Exercises. They incorporate a variety of strengthening and stretching exercises designed to promote strength, flexibility, coordination to improve the posture and alignment of the body. They work towards a toned body with healthy malleable muscles, releasing tensions and toxins, and allowing energy to flow and vitality to flourish.

UNDERSTANDING THE BASICS

Many fitness programmes focus on the development of muscles with the aim of creating an attractive physique, but although the end result can look good, it serves little useful purpose. Such body conditioning programmes concentrate mostly on muscle-strengthening. As a muscle is strengthened, it is contracted and becomes pumped up. A muscle that is continually contracted becomes shortened, solid and prone to injury.

On the other hand, if we look at the bodies of dancers, climbers, or practitioners of martial arts, they tend to be strong and yet be of slim build. These different disciplines require lithe, efficient, malleable muscles, which are developed through constant strengthening and complementary stretching work. For a muscle to be balanced and efficient, it needs to be worked in both directions, in other words by being contracted (shortened) and extended (lengthened). The layers of the muscle and tendons need to be able to glide freely over each other to enable us to move with ease. This mobility ensures that the muscle is able to respond to any eventuality and is protected against sudden pulling and subsequent injury. The muscle then becomes a clear channel, allowing a free flow of nutrients and energy through it and enabling potentially damaging toxins and waste products to be cleared away.

Joints and bones that receive a free flow of nutrients and energy via the surrounding muscles are better able to renew themselves. When tension in the muscles is released, the joints and bones are not held so tightly together and thus wear and tear of the joints is reduced. The wellbeing of the whole body is enhanced by this complementary strengthening and stretching approach.

The Daily Energy Exercises are based on this approach and have been developed from exercises used to train dancers. Dance exercises aim to create long, toned, relaxed muscles, capable of any movement. The exercises are devised so that one muscle group is first contracted and strengthened and then immediately stretched, either within the same exercise or in the next.

Strengthening

The strengthening exercises in this programme use only the natural weight of the body or limbs. I do not believe in using external weights for two reasons. Firstly, I find lifting weights unnatural. It puts a greater strain on the joints and ligaments, and it is very difficult to get a flow to the movements and not to jerk them. Secondly, once you start to use weights, you need to continue to use them on a regular basis if you are to maintain the progress you have made, and you may not always have access to weights or a gym. The Energy Source exercises are deliberately self-contained so that they can be done anywhere – at home, in the office, or in a hotel room.

All the exercises in this programme coordinate the movement with the breathing. The most important aspect of the breathing is the 'out' breath. When we are concentrating hard and exerting ourselves we often forget to breathe out, tending to hold our breath, thus retaining toxins in the muscles. This eventually leads to a build-up of toxins, which can result in headaches, muscle stiffness and low energy levels. By focusing our attention on the 'out' breath and keeping it firm and steady, we help disperse the toxins and other waste products.

The strengthening exercises use the inward and outward flow of the breath to increase their efficiency. The movements are coordinated so that the most strenuous moments of the exercise take place during the outward flow of the 'out' breath. Focusing on a fluid, continuous movement of the breath lengthens the muscles even as they are strengthening, ensuring that the muscles work with the minimum amount of tension and constriction and allowing blood and energy to flow through them.

For example, in the Curl Up exercise on page 102, which is a stomach strengthening exercise, the upper back curls up forwards off the floor from a lying position, led by the crown of the head, while the arms reach forwards. This curl up action engages all of the main abdominal muscle, which tenses and contracts very easily. The curl up is done with a sustained, conscious 'out' breath, imagining that breath and energy are flowing down and out through the body, and forwards and out through the raised arms. This outward flow of breath causes the abdominal muscles to release and open, ultimately developing a much deeper strength. The 'in' breath is then used as the spine uncurls to the floor, to inflate and relax the muscles that have been working. It is also used to support the release of a strengthening movement, so that the body does not collapse suddenly after the exertion. In the Curl Up exercise, the 'in' breath is used to control the rolling down of the spine to the floor, it keeps the movement smooth and fluid and prevents a giving in and collapse, thus helping to strengthen the body more.

In addition to integrating the breathing with the movement, many of the strengthening exercises use images of resistance. The images encourage one set of muscles to work against another set so that we literally use our own strength and imagination to strengthen ourselves. This type of exercise is known as isometric. The mechanics of the exercise may look simple, but the focus and attention on the image makes the exercise very powerful. You yourself are totally in control of how much or how little force to apply. Start gently with these exercises as they are deceptively simple, begin with few repetitions. Each strengthening exercise in the Daily Energy Programme has an individual explanation of the images involved. A good example is the very simple Half Knee Bends exercise on page 50.

Stand with your heels together and your toes as far apart as is comfortable. Now simply bend and straighten your knees without raising your heels off the floor. Keep your knees pointing directly over your toes at all times. The mechanics of this movement are easy and not particularly strengthening.

Now, try the same thing again, using the following image. Slowly bend your knees and imagine that you are pushing against a heavy, resistant wall with your knees, to the left side and to the right side. Move slowly, and this time you will feel a lot of resistance. It has now become a very powerful exercise.

To straighten your legs, change the image. Imagine you are squeezing a beach ball or pillow between your legs. Again move slowly. Resist straightening your legs until the very last moment as the knees come together. Exhausting isn't it? Here you are using two opposing sets of muscles – the inner and outer thighs – simultaneously. This is extremely strengthening and yet seemingly very gentle. Focusing on the quality of the movement at all times is essential for the effectiveness of this kind of exercise.

Stretching

As with the strengthening exercises, the most effective way of stretching is one that coordinates the movement with the breathing. Stretching dislodges toxins from the body and it is important that these are removed efficiently. Using a conscious, rhythmic breathing pattern while stretching focuses our attention and helps clear the muscles of toxins and stiffness.

Before going into a stretch, always take a moment to check that your body is correctly aligned and your weight evenly balanced. In the standing position, your weight should be centred on both feet, and if you are sitting make sure it is directly central, down through the spine and vertebrae.

The stretches in this programme use only the natural weight of the limbs and body and are never forced. Always approach a stretch gently, never vigorously. Breathe in as you prepare to stretch, elongating the spine and lifting your torso up out of the joints. As you reach up or over into the stretch, send the breath out firmly and release the body in the direction of the stretch. Use the outward flow of the 'out' breath to elongate you even more and try to imagine that your limbs are very long. Do not see the 'out' breath as a collapse – it is full of energy. Feel the energy flowing out through the stretch, way beyond your body into your energy field. Reach out or over to flow with it. As you breathe out firmly, imagine the breath leaving the body through all the five points of The Star simultaneously (see page 13), taking with it all kinds of unwanted toxins and clearing and releasing any energy blocks and stiffness in the muscles.

There are two different stretching techniques used within this programme. The first is a gentle method, good for impenetrable muscle groups that have been habitually held tense for some time. This method uses very small bounces in the direction of the stretch. Use only the relaxed weight of the limb or body to make tiny bouncing movements. Do not use any force to bounce the body. For example in 'Side Stretch' (page 57) as you reach the arm up and over to the side, control the 'out' breath and, with the weight of your upper body, take four or five gentle bounces over into the stretch. Then release the stretch and allow your upper body to rise up a little with the 'in' breath. Imagine drawing the 'in' breath into the muscles and expanding and releasing the area. Then, as you breathe out and gently bounce, see the 'out' breath clearing and dissipating any tension. Allow the natural weight of the limbs and body to take you a little further each time you stretch, but do not exert any pressure to push the stretch further.

The second technique is a more intense, sustained stretching method that is good for new or unexpected stiffness. Breathe in, to prepare to stretch, then lengthen the body and go into the stretch as you breathe out. Feel the breath coursing along the limbs and out of the body, escaping through the five points of The Star. Let the 'out' breath lengthen the body and then release into the muscles in one smooth movement. Now, breathe in and stay exactly where you are. Imagine drawing the 'in' breath into the muscles, expanding them and creating light and space within. Then breathe out strongly and release a little more in the direction of the stretch. Let your body flow with the outward-going breath and energy. On each 'out' breath, release further into the stretch, and on each 'in' breath, create more space within the muscles. Choose the technique that you feel most comfortable with. You may find different exercises feel better with a different technique. For very solid or contracted muscles, use the first technique and to work a muscle and increase flexibility, use the second.

As you stretch you will come to a natural point of resistance in the muscles. Do not push beyond this point, but imagine that you can draw breath into the very point of resistance. If you can, imagine a sensation like a yawn occurring in the muscle. To give you an idea of this sensation, create a yawn in your throat. The space that you feel in the back of your throat is the sensation you want to create in the muscle. Feel the point of resistance give a little as you 'yawn' in the muscle and breathe out.

When coming out of a stretch, always release it carefully. Each stretch in this programme has its own instructions on the most gentle way to do this. As a general rule, you should always 'roll out' of a stretch. So, if you are standing, curve your spine over, rolling it forwards, and then use an 'in' breath to inflate the spine and come to the upright position. If you are lying on the floor, roll onto your right side, curving your back around your knees in a foetal position, then push up onto your knees, uncurl the spine with an 'in' breath and come up to standing. Once in a comfortable position, shake out or rub the muscles you have just stretched.

For the first couple of weeks you may experience stiffness or a dull pain as new muscles get used. Try to work through this dull pain, by releasing further into the stretch on the 'out' breath and creating more space within the muscles on the 'in' breath, and it will soon pass. Continue with the Daily Energy Exercises but spend most time on the warm-up exercises and include lots of stretching work in your exercise sessions until the new stiffness passes. It would also be a good time to use the Energy Fountain preparatory exercises, particularly The Star and The Shooting Star, as these will help to clear general stiffness and release the muscles.

Should you experience a sharp pull or pain, stop, come out of the stretch gently and consult a medical practitioner. Never stretch or exercise beyond the natural point of resistance in the muscle. Be sensitive to your body's capabilities and gently work with them. Your body will know if an exercise feels too much or is simply not right for you. So always listen to your body and heed its advice.

Initially as you begin to practise the Daily Energy Exercises, there will seem an awful lot to concentrate on and many different sensations and images to hold in your Mind's Eye at the same time. With practice, this will happen automatically without any conscious thinking on your part. Eventually, you will be able to hold an image of your whole body in your Mind's Eye and at the same time be aware of the direction and flow of the energy and breath within a specific movement and to focus on its quality.

HOW TO USE THE DAILY ENERGY PROGRAMME

The Daily Energy Exercises are divided into five easy-to-follow steps as follows:

Step 1 Warming up
Step 2 Upper body
Step 3 Lower body
Step 4 Strengthening
Step 5 Stretching

Step 1 provides gentle warm up exercises that relax and loosen the muscles and joints, increase blood and oxygen supply to the whole body, helping prepare the body for action and preventing injury.

Step 2 focuses intensely on the upper body. The exercises involve strengthening and stretching movements that work on releasing and toning the arms, waist, shoulders, neck and upper back.

Step 3 takes the focus onto the lower body, these are strengthening and stretching movements that work and shape the legs, bottom and increase mobility in the hips, knees and ankles.

Step 4 is the most powerful step, it now unites the whole body and presents predominantly strengthening exercises that work the large muscle groups of the entire body, the back, stomach and pelvis.

Step 5 is a series of whole body stretches and relaxations to relieve stiffness and tension and to elongate the large muscle groups exercised in step 4.

Within these five steps you will find a wide variety of exercises to choose from so that you can respond to the different needs of your body at different times. During any one exercise session you can choose as many exercises as you wish from each step, depending on how much time you have available on that particular day, but always make sure you choose at least one exercise from each step. It's important that you perform the exercises in the order of the steps. The only exception to this rule is that you may alternate the exercises from Steps 4 and 5 so that you follow a strengthening exercise with an appropriate stretch, but always finish your session with a stretch from Step 5.

It's up to you whether you choose to spend most of your time working on the upper or lower body exercises or strengthening or stretching in any one session, or whether you work equally in all five steps.

The Daily Energy Programme

I tend to alternate the emphasis daily. One day I spend more time on the upper body than the lower body, then the next day I switch the emphasis. Ideally, the more time you have available to exercise, the more time you should spend focusing on the breathing, the quality of the movement and on the energy flow, since this will increase the effectiveness of all the exercises.

Within each step the exercises are arranged so that you can progress to the next exercise easily and safely. The earlier exercises are relatively gentle, and they gradually become more complex and strenuous as you work your way through the step. The more strenuous ones are marked with an asterisk, and these should only be attempted if you have already done one or more of the gentler exercises that appear earlier in that step.

To help initially with your choice of exercises, at the end of this chapter I have included some sample 20–30 minute programmes to suit varying needs. If you wish, you can try one of these at first and then begin to add or eliminate exercises according to your individual preference. Your selection is unlikely to be a fixed thing, but it may be helpful to choose a 20–30 minute programme of exercises, do them for a month and then to change and gradually introduce some new exercises. In addition, I have included suggestions for exercises which can be done in a five- or ten-minute break at the office or sitting at your desk, plus suggestions for exercises that can be done in a confined space when travelling.

Before you embark on an exercise, always read through the instructions first so that you get a sense of the general shape and intention of the exercise. Some of the more strenuous exercises have explanations on how to get into and also come out of the exercise safely. Follow these instructions and do not be tempted to cut them short and come out of an exercise abruptly. Getting into and out of an exercise is the time when most injuries are likely to occur. For this reason, where possible, try to choose a time to do the exercises when you will not be interrupted.

The exercises involve several different layers – breathing, movement, rhythm and direction of energy. You will not be able to take in all of these details and ideas in one go. Just let the ideas and images come together gradually as you become familiar with the exercise. The number of repetitions given is only a guideline. Listen to your own body – it will let you know if you are doing too few or too many.

Listening In

Before you begin your daily programme, take a moment to 'listen in' to your body. Stand in a relaxed position with your feet as wide apart as your hips and take four or five steady breaths. Focus on your breathing and try to get a general impression of how your body is feeling. This might be something like: 'generally tense' or 'rather weak and low in energy'; 'full of vitality' or 'agitated and nervous'; or 'very calm and still'. Breathe again and take your Mind's Eye into your body in the way that you did in the preparatory Energy Fountain exercises in Chapter 1. Be aware of any particular areas that feel blocked, tense, dark or impenetrable. Try to choose exercises that work on these particular areas and, as you exercise, consciously send your focus into these areas. Try to gently coax them open with the breath and the movements and allow the energy images to flow freely through them.

If your whole body feels tense when you 'listen in', then try to choose exercises which are generally energizing and clearing. If your body feels 'calm and still' or 'full of vitality' or 'very open and free of tension', then simply choose whichever exercises you enjoy doing. There is no better guide than to work intuitively at this point. Remember that you will know what is best for your own body and that all the answers are within you, if you listen. Don't do anything that does not feel right for you. Choose the exercises and movements that suit you or your mood on that particular day. This will become easier over time as you become familiar with the range of exercises.

At first you'll find it easier to identify the movements or exercises that are not right for you. You will feel this quite strongly. Certain exercises may feel uncomfortable, or you may simply dislike them. Avoid these exercises for the time being, and try coming back to them at a later date, as your sensations may change over time.

Many of the exercises begin with a preparatory check through the body to make sure that your alignment is correct and to remind you to release unnecessary tensions. This is an extension of the 'listening in' process which really goes on all the time you are exercising and moving.

The process of continuously removing unwanted tension by listening in and then consciously visualizing free-flowing energy through the body is what will make your daily exercising more effective and increase your actual energy and vitality.

Breathing

Strong breathing is fundamental to energy flow, vitality and wellbeing and so is a central focus of the exercises. A strong breathing pattern that is in harmony with your movement acts like bellows, drawing and guiding the Universal Energy throughout the body.

The Daily Energy Exercises combine the rising and falling of the breath with the natural rhythm of the movement of the body. You will find that this combination will help you overcome many of the strenuous points within an exercise where you might otherwise use unnecessary effort and tension. These exercises will develop your awareness of breathing and encourage confident, conscious breathing that strengthens the action of the breath.

Try not to force your breathing, but aim for a continuous motion of the breath where the moment of turn-around between the outward and the inward flow is almost imperceptible. When we are tense we have a tendency to hold onto our breath or to breathe out shallowly, causing us to hold onto toxins. Try to make the 'out' breath a conscious clearing out of the lungs. After a conscious 'out' breath, the 'in' breath will come as a natural reaction.

The rhythm of the movement is also an

important aspect of the exercises, so try to find a confident rhythm that coordinates your movement with your breathing. Whether you are circling, swinging or stretching, the rhythm should feel good and the exercise beautiful and pleasurable to do. Never jerk or force movements, but keep them fluid. The gentle circling that is part of many of the exercises is a good way of warming up, since it massages the muscles and joints, gently coaxing them to work. Should you feel any stiffness, rub or massage the muscles before and after an exercise to encourage them to release the tension.

Once you begin to exercise on a regular basis you may start to notice almost daily variations in your energy levels and in the state of your muscles. This is because the body acts as a very sensitive barometer to your state of mind, sleep patterns, activities, emotions, stress levels and diet. Even after weeks of feeling supple and physically good, you may suddenly experience days of stiffness. If this occurs, simply coax the body and gently work through the stiffness, focusing the breath into the relevant areas, and make sure you include a lot of stretching work in your sessions. The stiffness will eventually disappear. In addition, you could try doing one session a week of the Energy Fountain preparatory exercises in Chapter 1. This will help you become aware of the areas of your body that need strengthening or releasing and keep the energy images and sensations fresh in your Mind's Eye.

Be patient with your body. It is an organism in a constant state of flux as it tries to cope with everything you demand of it. Your progress in your exercise programme may not always be linear, but by developing the skills to 'listen in' to your body, your ability to respond to and deal with any changes will improve rapidly, enabling you to stay balanced and improving your general health and wellbeing. If you are overweight or below the recommended weight for your size, you may find that your body finds its natural weight as you develop a greater sensitivity to its needs and as a result of the increased energy flow. Stubborn fat deposits may be dissipated as these areas of the body are opened and the toxins are flushed through.

Where to practise

Try to choose a peaceful part of your home in which to exercise. Make sure it is warm enough, with fresh air circulating through and, ideally, with a view to focus on. If this is not possible, have something beautiful, uplifting and inspirational in the room such as a bowl of fresh flowers, a plant or a candle, something you can focus on while you are exercising. When I'm travelling I always carry with me a shell from my home or a photograph of my favourite mountains. You could use a crystal, a flower or even a glass of sparkling clear mineral water. You will also need a towel or mat to place on the floor, plus a chair or a wall to use as support.

When to practise

Choose a suitable time of the day for your exercise session, whatever time is easiest and most comfortable for you. I prefer to exercise as part of my morning get-up routine, since I find that this clears my mind and my body and sets up my energy level and focus for the day. This has become such a natural start to the day for me now that if I were to miss an exercise session, it would feel as strange as forgetting to have breakfast.

If the morning is not convenient or simply unimaginable, try exercising in your lunch-hour at work. If you do this before eating, it will help clear away the stresses of the morning, quieten your mind, which will help you solve any problems that may have arisen in the morning while refreshing your body for the afternoon. Exercising just before bedtime aids digestion as it increases blood and oxygen flow and distribution of nutrients and also aids the action of the intestines. It helps the body rid itself of toxins that have accumulated during the day and, providing you do not choose the most energizing exercises, relaxes the mind and body, ensuring a good night's sleep.

What to wear

It's entirely up to you what you wear when you exercise, but avoid wearing tight clothing and take off any jewellery, watches, belts or ties that are potentially hazardous. I prefer to wear loose, comfortable exercise clothes – it's best if you don't have to think what to wear every time. Some people choose to exercise without clothes. However, I find that being dressed helps to keep any thoughts or distractions concerning my body at bay and allows me to focus

on enjoying the intention of the movement and the energy. It's very important that your body is warm enough though, particularly your feet, as they form an essential connection to the the earth. Work in bare feet, or in socks if your feet are cold.

To finish

The Wave Breathing exercise from Chapter 1 is an excellent way to round off your exercise session. After exercising, take a moment to thank your body. Thank it for all its years of service to you and acknowledge the fact that you have put aside this time for yourself. Above all, enjoy feeling your body open and stretch.

Whenever possible, complement your daily exercise with other forms of gentle aerobic activity such as walking, swimming or cycling. These activities are known as low impact aerobics. They have aerobic benefits, but involve only a limited amount of shock to the joints and vertebrae. Aerobic activity increases heart and lung capacity and improves circulation and general stamina. It is currently thought that for exercise to have aerobic benefits it must raise your pulse rate above its normal level and maintain that raised level for more than 20 minutes. Although the emphasis of the Daily Energy Exercises is on stretching and toning the body and on vitality and general wellbeing, the exercises can also be used to aerobic benefit. Once you are familiar with them you can perform them without pausing for a 20-30 minute session.

Each exercise session should leave you feeling uplifted and refreshed. The image of Universal Energy coursing through the body like wonderful, constant, self-replenishing water, working in harmony with your breathing, has the power to release and transform the body. Take what works for you from The Energy Source and begin to incorporate it into your life; leave the rest.

DAILY ENERGY SOURCE EXERCISES

STEP ONE
Warm Up/Whole Body

1. Swing, bounce & shift
2. Upward reach
3. Hula hoop hip circles
4. Curl-down
5. Skiing swing
6. Forward scoop
7. Side scoop
8. Sitting bounces
9. *Spiral swing
10. *Gathering & opening
11. *Upper body circling
12. *Half & full knee bends
13. *Bounce & leg stretch
14. *Drawing energy

STEP TWO
Upper Body

1. Toxin release
2. Side stretch
3. Concentric circles
4. Elbow press
5. Hand & arm circles
6. Wings
7. *Arm press
8. *Flamenco contract & open
9. *Towel stretch
10. *Shoulder chair stretch

STEP THREE
Lower Body

1. Foot strengthener
2. Flex & push
3. Leg brushes
4. Heel raisers
5. Zen leg lifts
6. Front of thigh
7. Flex & stretch
8. Foot bounce & circle
9. Outer thigh chair press
10. Inner thigh chair press
11. *Knee lifts
12. *Figure of eight
13. *Travelling knee lifts
14. *Hip Flexor
15. *Sitting side stretch
16. *Sitting flex

* An asterisk denotes a more strenuous exercise. These should only be attempted if you have already done one or more of the gentler exercises that appear earlier in that step.

Preparation: *Listening in*

STEP FOUR Strengthening	STEP FIVE Stretching
1. Cycling	1. 'All fours' curve & stretch
2. Spiral slide	2. Spine breathing
3. Curl up	3. Crossed leg stretch
4. Shoulder stand: cycling	4. Upper back breathing
Shoulder stand: twist	5. Back alignment
Shoulder stand: scissors	6. Diagonal shoulder stretch
Shoulder stand: isometric	7. Hip stretch
5. 'All fours' leg lifts	8. Thigh stretch
6. Leg circles	9. *Wave stretch
7. *Swing your weight	10. *'Over the top' spine release
8. *Twister	11. *Spiral stretch
9. *Pelvic push up	12. *Diagonal reach
10. Pelvic lift	13. *Chair stretch
11. *'On the walk' lifts	
12. *Pelvic tilt	
13. *Glutaeus Maximus	To finish: **Wave breathing**

STEP 1

WARMING UP

1 SWING, BOUNCE AND SHIFT

A gentle warm-up exercise that is particularly useful if you are feeling stiff or generally rough.

Preparation

* Stand in the centre of your exercise space with your feet relaxed on the floor, about as wide apart as your hips. Relax your arms by your sides.
* If you have time, pass your Mind's Eye through your body as in the Standing Light preparatory exercise (see page 12) and release any tension or gripping in the muscles.
* Bend your knees a little and begin.

Sequence

* First, start a rhythmic forward and backward swinging movement with both arms. This movement should be fairly energetic, so keep the size of the swing fairly small.
* Second, allow the weight of the arms and upper body to create a bounce in the knees each time you swing forwards or back. Do not straighten the knees at all – just let the bounce deepen the bend in the knees. Imagine your arms and hands are very heavy. Use the swing and bounce to release any tension in the large muscle groups – the shoulders and neck; the small of the back and the hips; the jaw, throat and face.
* Third, slowly begin to shift the weight of the body onto your right foot as you bounce and swing. Take about six bounces to transfer all your weight onto the foot. Bounce on the right foot for a moment and

then take six bounces to transfer all the weight back in the other direction onto the left foot. Bounce on the left foot for a moment. The transfer of weight should gently massage the feet on the floor and help to relax them (fig. below). Keep going, transferring your weight from foot to foot, and continue until you feel the tension release.

Notes
* Establish one movement first before adding the next. Once you have built up to all three, keep going as long as feels pleasurable. The longer you continue, the more tension you will release.

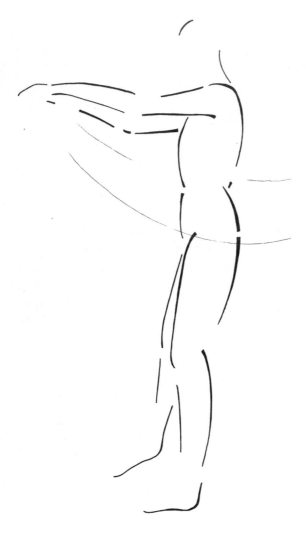

2 UPWARD REACH

A general warm-up and energizing stretch that elongates the sides of the body.

Preparation
* Stand with your feet a little wider apart than your hips. Spread and relax the feet on the floor.
* Open your arms wide to the sides and breathe for a moment using the image of the Open Star (see page 13), drawing the energy in through the feet, arms and head on the 'in' breath and sending it out through the five points on the 'out' breath.
* Breathe in and raise both arms up over your head, release the shoulders, and begin.

Sequence
* Breathe out and bend the right knee, pushing into the floor as deeply as you can, and shift all your weight onto the right foot. At the same time, reach upwards with the right arm and hand, directing the 'out' breath and energy up through the fingers out into the universe and also down through the leg into the earth. As you

breathe out and send the energy in both directions, feel that you are creating space in the centre of your body (fig. below).

* Breathe out, bend your left knee and push deep into the floor with the left foot. At the same time, reach upwards with the left arm and hand. Send the breath and energy out through the fingers and down through the leg into the earth. Be aware of the stretch in the centre of the body.

* As you breathe in, release the stretch. Push away from the floor with the left foot, shift your weight onto your right leg and continue as before.

* Repeat about ten times in total, shifting your weight rhythmically left and right in a rocking motion.

Notes

* Imagine that you are pushing down through a resistant material as you shift your weight. Move smoothly through the feet. This shifting movement should feel strong yet fluid.

* As you reach upwards with the arm and press down into the floor with the legs, be aware of sending energy in both directions. You will feel an elongation in the waist and ribs. Try to elongate the centre of the body further with each shift of the weight. Find your own rhythm that coordinates your breathing with the shifting of the weight.

* Breathe in and release the stretch, but leave the arm above your head, and shift your weight onto your left foot.

3 HULA HOOP HIP CIRCLES

This is a really good relaxation and warm-up exercise for the whole body. If you can relax into the exercise, it will massage the upper body, shoulders and neck.

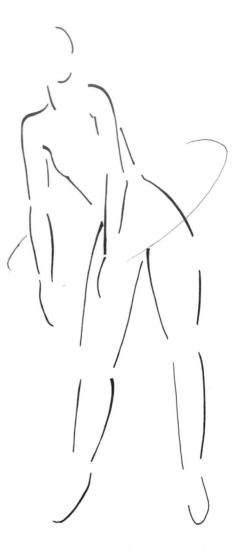

Preparation

* Stand with your feet slightly wider apart than your hips, bend the knees and keep your spine upright.
* Release your upper body, allowing your arms and shoulders to go heavy and to drop away from the neck. With an 'out' breath, release the ribcage.

Sequence

* Begin to circle the hips in one direction. Let them drop forwards, to the side, to the back and to the other side. Again forwards, side, back in a continuous circle. Make the circles as large as possible, moving the hips as far away from the centre of the body as you can. Keep the rest of the upper body – the head, arms, shoulders – heavy and relaxed and allow them to swing around in response to the movement of your hips (fig. right).
* After about six to eight rotations, start to make the circles smaller, then change direction and circle the hips to the other side. Keep the rest of the body relaxed. Try not to hold it or carry it. Just let the rest of the body follow naturally as you change the direction of the hips.

* Try about six to eight large circles in each direction, then repeat. Gradually reduce the size of the circles in order to change direction each time.

4 CURL DOWN

This is a very gentle exercise to animate and stretch the spine, using only the breath and the weight of the body.

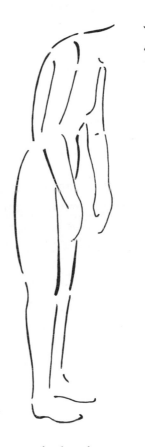

Preparation

* Stand with your feet as wide apart as your hips. Relax the feet and let them spread on the floor. Unlock the knees.
* Breathe for a moment using the image of the Energy Fountain (see page 13), allowing the image to lift and elongate your spine and create space in the back of the neck and head.

Sequence

* Holding onto those sensations, breathe out and tilt the head forwards. Breathe in, then on the next 'out' breath, curl the spine over about one vertebra. Continue like this so that on each 'out' breath, you release over forwards one vertebra. Try to be aware of each vertebra as you slowly curl down towards the floor. Feel each one open and release as gravity and the weight of the body draws it down. Release the back of the neck and let the arms and shoulders simply hang down. Keep your feet and knees relaxed (fig. top right).
* When you have gone as far over as is comfortable, on one long 'in' breath, draw yourself up to the upright position, inflating and uncurling the spine vertebra by vertebra and placing the vertebrae one on top of the other like building blocks.

* Breathe out as the head returns to the top of the spine, relaxing the shoulders and arms.
* Repeat about two or three times. Each time you curl down, you should be able to elongate the spine and release a little more.

Notes

* Try to maintain the Energy Fountain image throughout the exercise. When your spine is curled over, the energy that is coming out of the top of your head will also be directed back into the earth.

Curl Down Variation

This variation further increases the elong-ation of the spine.

* Go into the exercise as before. Curl over vertebra by vertebra, with each 'out' breath, as far as is comfortable.
* On a slow deliberate 'out' breath, bend your knees as deeply as you can without lifting your heels from the floor. Direct the breath down your spine, out through the top of your head and into the floor. Allow your body to fold over the knees and let the shoulders and arms hang down heavy. Release the back of your neck and let your head simply hang (fig. below).

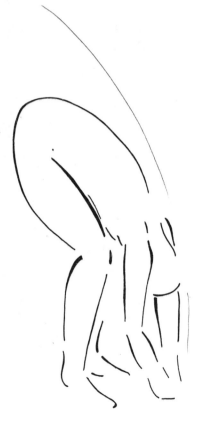

* On an 'in' breath, draw the breath in through the soles of the feet and inflate and slowly straighten the legs. As you do this, try to leave the upper body where it is, thereby elongating the spine.
* Repeat three or four times. With each 'out' breath, bend the knees and fold the body further over the legs, and with each 'in' breath, leave the head and chest where they are, inflate and straighten the legs to elongate the spine further.
* To come out of the exercise, on one firm 'in' breath uncurl the spine vertebra by vertebra until the head returns to the upright position.

Notes
* You may experience a vertebra 'pop' or release while you are doing this exercise. This is nothing to worry about. It is the joint releasing a vacuum.

5 SKIING SWING

An energetic whole body warm-up exercise which increases the circulation and release toxins.

Preparation
* Stand in the centre of your exercise space with your arms down by your sides.
* Breathe in right down to the stomach and then with a deliberate 'out' breath empty the lungs. Shake your arms and shoulders

to send the air and the toxins from your body and into the earth.

* Breathe again and empty your lungs and your body by shaking out your arms and shoulders as before.

Sequence

* Breathe in and raise both arms up in front of you then carry them up over your head (fig. below).
* With the 'out' breath, swing the arms and the torso forwards. Reach out with the arms, sending energy out through the arms as you swing down, curving your head and spine and bending your knees. The deepest part of the bend should be as the arms swing down and point directly into the floor.

* As the arms carry on and swing up behind the body, breathe in and lift up a little but keep your head and spine curved over your bent legs (fig. below).

* Without pausing, breathe out and reverse the swing. Swing your arms forwards. As they swing down towards the floor, allow the knees to bend deeper, then swing the arms up in front of you.

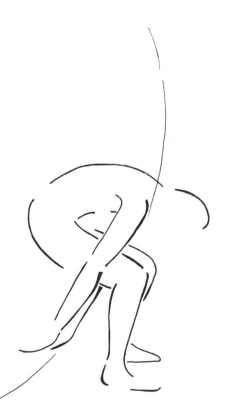

* Breathe in and straighten your legs, bringing the arms directly over your head.
* Breathe out and circle both arms back behind the body and down by your sides.
* Breathe in and continue to circle the arms, bringing them up in front of you and directly over your head.
* Breathe out, bend the elbows and relax the hands and forearms so that they drop backwards behind your head, elbows pointing upwards. Open your chest and turn the chest and head up towards the ceiling slightly and gently press the elbows towards each other. Take care to control the backwards movement of the head. It should lean back only as a natural continuation of the spine in response to the opening of the chest to the ceiling.
* Now, start the whole sequence again. Breathing in, straighten the arms and reach way up above your head with your arms.
* Breathe out and swing the arms and body forwards, bending your knees and curving your spine over the knees.
* Breathe in as the arms swing behind you and lift your body a little.
* Breathe out and reverse the direction by swinging the arms forwards.
* Breathe in and straighten your legs and body, bringing your arms above your head.
* Breathe out and circle the arms behind you.
* Breathe in as you carry the circle on in front and then up above your head.
* Breathe out and drop your forearms down behind your head, gently pressing the elbows together and opening the chest.
* Try ten swings in total, finishing with the arms above the head. Lower the arms slowly, then breathe out and stand still for

a moment before going on to your next exercise.

Notes

* This exercise really generates a lot of energy. Imagine the arms extend far away from you, and feel the weight of your arms and upper body as you release them into the swing. Their weight generates a lot of power as you swing.
* Let the energy and swing of the movements dictate the rhythm of your breathing rather than the other way round. The 'out' breath uses the weight of the body in the swing and is always coordinated with a downward releasing movement. The 'in' breath inflates and lifts the body each time.
* Throughout the exercise, take care not to collapse totally. Stay lifted and supported in the stomach, as if someone had their arms around your waist and were supporting some of the weight of your body. This image is very helpful as it gives you a strong centre to swing from and allows your spine and shoulders to stretch away from your centre. It also prevents you from falling off balance.

6 FORWARD SCOOP

A rhythmic warm-up exercise for the spine that increases energy flow and circulation.

Preparation

* Stand with your toes pointing forwards, feet parallel and as wide apart as your hips.
* Bend both knees equally, keeping your heels on the floor. Relax the thigh muscles.
* Start with both arms bent and elbows lifted so that the arms are at shoulder height and the palms of the hands are facing the chest.

Sequence

* Draw the right elbow back behind the body and allow your spine to spiral so that you are facing the right side. Keep your knees and hips facing front as much as possible. Now unfold the arm, extending it behind you.
* Breathe out and scoop your right arm wide to the side and then forwards at shoulder height, leading with the palm of the hand, palm facing forwards. Imagine you are pressing a body of water or air away with the curve of your arm. Reach far away from the body. As you scoop forwards, allow the momentum of the movement to bounce you deeper in the legs (fig. right).
* Breathe in and bounce up again naturally as the arm reaches the front. The movement of the right arm will cause the spine to spiral and face the left side. As the spine spirals to the left, draw your left elbow backwards directly behind the body and uncurl the arm behind you. Let the right arm bend in towards the chest, with the elbow lifted at shoulder height.
* Breathe out forcefully and scoop the left arm wide to the side and then forwards, exactly as you did with the right arm, lead-

ing with the palm of the hand. Keep the image of shifting a mass of water or air with the curve of your arm and let the knees bounce deeper with the momentum of the scoop.
* Breathe in as the left arm reaches the front and come up a little from the deep bounce. The body will naturally spiral to face the right side. As the spine spirals, bend your right arm in towards your chest

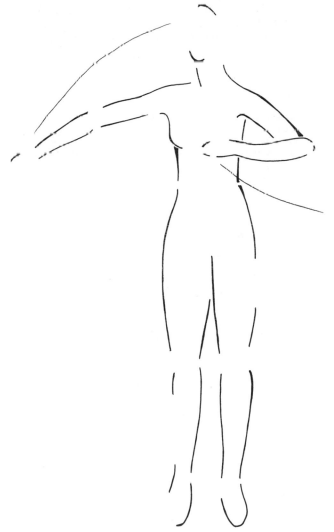

and take the right elbow back behind you, letting the left arm bend in towards the chest, elbow lifted at shoulder height.

* Try at least ten scoops, alternating sides.

Notes

* Notice that the movements of the left and right side of the body completely overlap each other and are coordinated. It should feel like some kind of inverse swimming motion.

* Try to make the movement rhythmic and fluid. Relax and let yourself be carried along with the energy and momentum of the scoop. Focus on sending the breath out deliberately on the forward scoop and let the 'in' breath simply be a natural reaction as you open the arm out behind you.

7 SIDE SCOOP

A rhythmic whole body warm-up.

Preparation

* Before you begin, bounce up and down on your heels for a few moments, and with a firm 'out' breath, shake out your arms, shoulders and upper body. Shake out any tension from your fingertips and release the upper body.

* Stand in the centre of your exercise space with your feet wider apart than your hips – about two feet (60cm) apart – and arms relaxed by your sides.

Sequence

* Begin with a rhythmic swaying motion that shifts the weight of the body from one foot to the other. As you shift the weight from one foot to the other, bend the knee deeply, pushing smoothly but powerfully into the floor. Keep the swaying movement even and steady. Now imagine that the sways are in groups of three – ie 'right, left, right', then 'left, right, left' and so on. Try this until you have the sensation of beginning with the right foot for three sways and then beginning with the left foot for three sways.

* Now add an arm movement. Beginning on a 'right, left, right' sway, as you shift your weight to the right, breathe out and arc your right arm up from the side of your body, leading with the back of the hand and taking the arm all the way up to above your head to reach a long way away from the body with the fingertips. This movement should feel like a scoop to the side (fig. right).

* Breathe in as you shift your weight onto your left leg, and curl the right arm straight down behind your head and behind the body to finish by your side (fig. far right).

* Breathe out and scoop the right hand to the right side again as you shift your weight onto the right foot. When the arm reaches about shoulder height, shift your focus immediately to the left arm and leave your right arm to curl down to your side by the most direct route.

* Without a pause in the swaying rhythm go straight into a 'left, right, left' sway by breathing in and shifting your weight onto your left foot, bending deeply and pressing

firmly into the floor on the left side. At the same time, scoop your left arm up in a wide arc to the side, swinging the arm way out to the side and then up above your head.

* Breathe out and shift your weight to the right. Curl your left arm directly down behind your head and body to finish by your side.

* Breathe in again and as you shift your weight onto your left foot, scoop your left

arm up to the left side, reaching far away from your body and leading with the back of the hand. Finish the scoop around shoulder height and, staying with the rhythm, shift your focus immediately to the right hand and let the left hand curl down to your side by the most direct route.

* Keep going, and try ten groups of 'threes' in total.

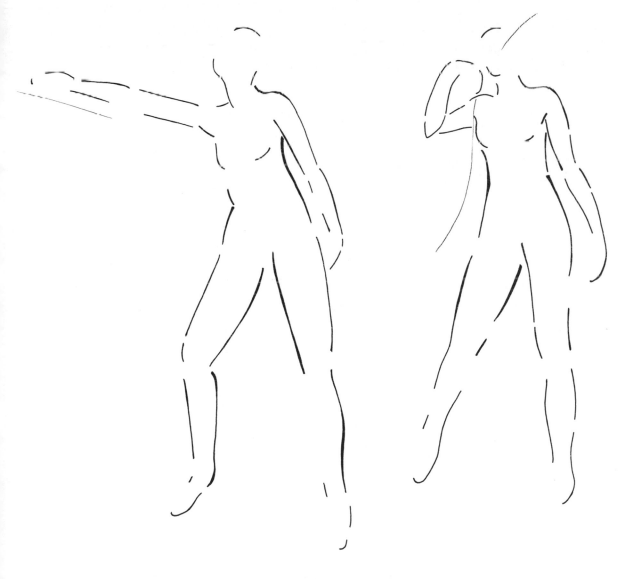

Notes

* When you are familiar with the movements, aim to keep the rhythm steady and fluid. Enjoy the scooping movement, reaching and stretching far out beyond the body. Try to feel the flow of the energy and the momentum.

* As you do the exercise, imagine you are guiding a ball playfully on the back of your hand. Guide the ball on the back of the right hand for three sways and, as you shift your focus to the opposite hand, throw the ball to the left hand, and then very dexterously guide it on the back of the left hand for three sways.

8 SITTING BOUNCES

A gentle exercise to warm up the spine, using coordinated breathing.

Preparation

* Sit on the floor on a mat or towel, with the soles of your feet together and legs relaxed. Let your knees drop outwards to the sides. Place your feet about two feet (60 m) away from your body. If this is not comfortable, then take them further away from the body and, if necessary, separate the soles of the feet a little, until you can sit upright in this position. Place your hands lightly on your ankles or calves.

* On a firm 'out' breath relax the shoulders, spine, legs and hips.

Sequence

* Take a very slow deliberate 'in' breath and imagine you are drawing energy into the body from the earth beneath you. As the energy travels up your spine, see it lifting and invigorating one vertebra after another. Feel it expanding and filling the space in the neck, then travelling up the back of the head, circling in the head cavity and escaping beyond your head. Draw the breath in continuously until your spine and head are lifted and upright (fig. below).

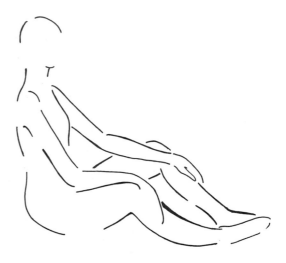

* Control the 'out' breath and imagine that the energy is slowly receding back down the spine into the earth, leaving the body and releasing the spine vertebra by vertebra. Allow your head and upper back to curve over towards your feet as the energy recedes.

* Stay curved over towards your feet. On the 'in' breath, bounce gently towards your feet for a count of four. Do not grip with your hands or pull yourself towards your

feet, but just use the relaxed weight of the body (fig. below).

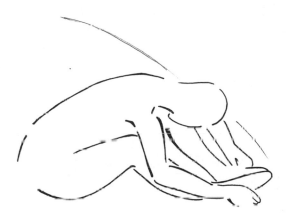

* As you breathe out, continue bouncing for a further four counts. Release into the muscles as you breathe out and allow the weight of your body to take you a little further towards your feet. Imagine your spine and neck long, and direct the breath out through the crown of your head, beyond your feet.
* From this curved-over position start the sequence again by filling and lifting the spine from the base with a slow deliberate 'in' breath. Slowly raise the spine vertebra by vertebra so that the neck and head are the last to uncurl, and continue as before.
* Repeat the whole four-breath pattern at least four times. Finish with the slow 'in' breath drawing you up to the upright position. Stay upright, breathe out naturally and relax your shoulders. Shake out your legs in front of you, rub your thighs, hips and the small of your back vigorously for a moment before going on to your next exercise.

*9 SPIRAL SWING

This whole body swing increases the mobility of the spine, the upper torso and tones the waist.

Preparation
* Stand with your feet parallel and as wide apart as your hips. Allow your arms to hang relaxed by your sides. Relax your shoulders, neck and jaw. Imagine that the whole of your back is in contact with a wall.
* Bend your knees and slide down the 'wall' a little, keeping your body upright and your weight centred between both feet.

Sequence
* The movement begins in the centre of your body. Keeping your knees and hips facing front, start to spiral your spine to one side. Let the head move naturally as an extension of the spine, and let the rest of the torso, the shoulders and then the arms follow in response to the movement of the spine so that you are facing the side.
* Now start to spiral to the other side, starting from the centre of the body and allowing the torso, shoulders and arms to follow as a natural reaction to the movement (fig. right).
* Repeat the spiralling movement from side to side until you have a rhythmic swing going. Keep your breathing natural, but try to coordinate it with the swinging motion. For example, you could breathe in smoothly over two spirals, filling and

43

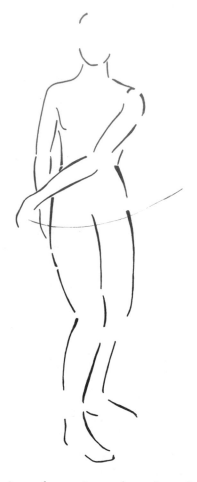

allow the head to be lightly placed on top of the spine. Keep the feet, knees and hips directly pointing forwards and not involved in the spiral. Release any gripping of the toes or rigidity in the thighs and knees. Maintain a fluidity in them by breathing out down through the legs, imagining water energy pouring through them back into the earth.

Spiral Swing Variation

This variation is very energizing as it combines the swing with the power of the legs to increase the energy flow. The body weight shifts from one foot to the other as you spiral, which increases the spiral and opens the body.

* Stand with your feet parallel, as wide apart as your hips, and release any tension. Place your spine against an imaginary wall and bend your knees.
* Breathe in as you start the spiral to your right side and raise the heel of your right foot slightly.
* With the 'out' breath, step out wide to the right side so that the feet are now much wider apart than the hips. Press down into the floor and bend the right knee deeply. Continue the spiral swing to the right with the upper body following as before (fig. right).
* Breathe in and begin the spiral to the other side, straightening the legs as you spiral. As you swing through centre and face the front, throw your arms and chest wide

elongating the spine, then breathe out smoothly over two spirals.
* Try 10–20 spiral swings in total. To come out of the exercise, gradually decrease the amount of energy and impetus in the spiral. You should come to a natural stop over two or three swings.

Notes

* As you swing and spiral around your spine try to be aware of the following. Keep your arms relaxed and hanging at all times. Try not to carry them. Relax the jaw and

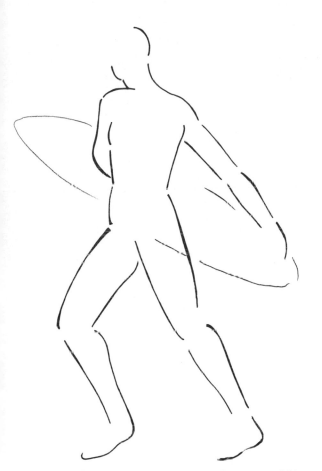

Notes

* Find your own rhythm for the swing, one that combines the powerful breathing and the opening and spiralling movements as you shift your weight left and right. Breathe out as you transfer your weight, pushing down into the floor and spiralling with the spine, then breathe in as you raise up and throw open the arms and chest into the Open Star position.

* The shifting movement of the legs and hips should feel strong and grounded, while the body opens, spirals and swings above.

* Keep your spine vertical over the hips and knees. Try not to let it collapse over the knee as you spiral to the side.

* Keep your feet, knees and hips pointing directly to the front. Resist the temptation to twist them with the energy of the swing to try and increase the movement.

open in the Open Star position (see page 13).
* On the 'out' breath, shift your weight onto your left foot, pressing down into the floor and bending your left knee, and continue the spiral around to face the left.
* Breathe in and straighten the legs as you start to spiral to the right, throwing the arms wide as you pass through centre.
* Try 10–20 spiral swings. Come out of the exercise over three or four swings, gradually decreasing the energy flowing through the movement.

*10 GATHERING AND OPENING

A whole body warm-up that gathers energy into the body.

Preparation

* Stand with your feet relaxed but firmly on the floor and as wide apart as your hips. Feel the whole of each foot in contact with the floor and be aware of the support that the floor is giving.

* Open the chest and open the arms wide to the sides. Breathe for a moment and open the body using the Open Star image (see page 13), breathing energy in through and then out of all five points.

Sequence

* With a strong 'out' breath, bend the knees and drop the upper body forwards in the direction of the feet (fig. below). This should feel like a complete release, as if you were a rag doll. Carry the arms down and scoop them together by your feet as if gath-

ering up energy. Maintain some support in the stomach area. Imagine someone is holding their arms around your waist to support you and your upper body is releasing over these imaginary arms (fig. below).

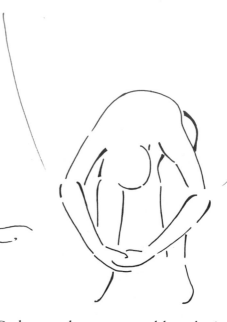

* Gather up the energy and breathe in. Let the energy enter through the soles of your feet, and use it to lift and straighten your legs and spine up to standing.
* As you straighten up, carry both arms up in front of your body and over your head, then separate them out to either side to the Open Star position.
* Breathe out and open the chest to the ceiling, allowing the head to go back just a little as a natural extension of the spine. At the same time, carry the arms across at shoulder height to meet each other in front so that the arms form a circle in front of your chest. This circle balances the upward and backward arch of the spine. Be aware that your open chest and the circle formed by your arms contain energy (fig. right).

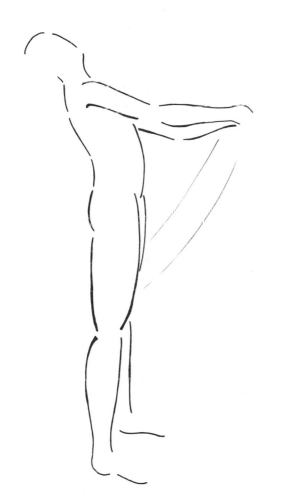

Notes

* This exercise has four distinct movements: drop forwards as you release the breath out; draw up as you breathe in; breathe out and open the chest to the ceiling, forming a circle in front of the chest with the arms; breathe in and straighten up. Try to find your own rhythm for the four movements so that they become one cycle that flows. Move with the breath, but always have a sense of carrying the body and arriving carefully into each position. Do not allow the body to just swing with its own weight.

*11 UPPER BODY CIRCLING

A warm-up exercise for the torso, waist, spine, shoulders and neck.

Preparation

* Stand in the centre of your exercise space, with your feet as wide apart as your hips and firmly planted on the floor. Rock your weight backwards and forwards a little until you are sure your weight is evenly distributed over both feet.

* Bend your knees, keeping your spine straight and long as if you were sitting on a chair. The lower body, from the waist down, should stay in this position throughout the exercise. Take care to keep the feet and the legs 'alive' and not to grip or hold

* With the 'in' breath, straighten up the spine and throw the arms wide to the sides into the starting position, ready to begin the sequence again by releasing forwards on the next 'out' breath.

* Try this sequence about five times at first and gradually work up to ten over the first few weeks. Finish on the 'in' breath at the end of the cycle, with the arms open wide to the sides. The increased energy, oxygen and blood flow may make you feel a little dizzy at first, so stand still and just breathe for a moment until this clears before going on to your next exercise.

energy in them by making them rigid. Breathe through the soles of your feet and imagine energy flowing into your lower body and out through the earth. Again, imagine someone is holding you firmly around the waist and supporting you. As you move your upper body in this exercise, the movement will take place over these imaginary arms.

* Breathe in and bring both arms up in front of you and curve them to form a circle, fingertips meeting in front of your chest and palms facing you. You are enclosing and carrying energy from your energy field with your arms. The arms should stay in this position throughout the exercise.

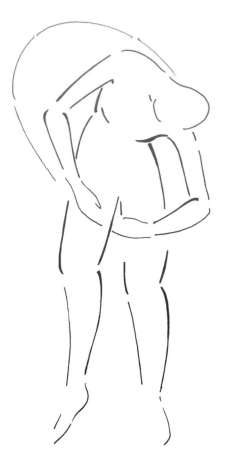

Sequence

* Breathe out and lean the weight of the upper body to the right. Roll your upper body forwards, curving the spine and the head, and then down over your bent legs. Without pausing, continue to roll to the left side (fig. top right).

* Breathe in and continue circling, using the breath to lift your upper body to the left side and then up to centre in the starting position. Keep the legs bent yet alive the whole time.

* Breathe out and start to reverse the direction of the roll. Lean over to the left, staying very strong in the waist and keeping your weight centred between your feet. Curve the spine and head forwards to the left side and then down over your bent legs. Continue the circle by rolling to the right.

* Breathe in and draw your torso up to the right side and then up to centre in the upright position.

* Repeat this sequence again, circling first to the right and then to the left.

* Now, over four breaths, circle without pausing as follows:

—Breathe out and circle to the right as before, curving over to the side, then forwards and rolling up to the left.

—Lift up to the left side on the 'in' breath, and pass through the upright position to continue the circle (fig. far right).

—Breathe out and circle to the right again, releasing your upper body and curving your spine and head forwards. Pause over your bent knees. You have completed one and a half circles.

—Breathe in and use the breath to

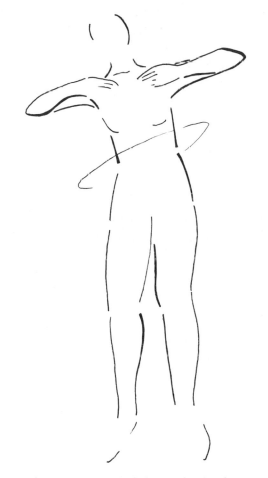

* Now breathe out and drop the body to the left side, roll and curve the spine forwards as before, then breathe in and circle on up to the right. Pass through the upright position again, then drop to the left and curve forwards with the 'out' breath. Finish the one and a half circles curved forwards over your bent knees.
* Breathe in and uncurl the spine, drawing the body upright with the incoming breath and pause.
* Try the whole sequence twice to the left and twice to the right. To finish, lower the arms and slowly straighten the legs. Shake out any tension in the arms, shoulders, feet and legs.

Notes

* The most important element of this exercise is the support around your waist by the imaginary arms. This keeps your torso stable and centred so that you are able to isolate the circling of the upper body without coming off balance. Once you feel secure in the centre of your body and confident that you are not going to lose your balance, you can begin to release your upper body more into the swing. Try to make the circles flow one into another to form a continuous movement pattern.

uncurl your spine and draw the body up to the upright position. If your legs and arms are tired at this point, straighten your legs and drop the arms and shake out any tension. Then resume the starting position. If you are not tense, just carry straight on.
* You are going to repeat the whole sequence from the beginning, starting your first circle to the left side. Breathe out and lean to the left, curve forwards over the legs, over to the right and then on the 'in' breath roll up to the right side and into the upright position. Roll to the right, completing a full circle. Repeat once more to each side.

*12 KNEE BENDS

An intense isometric warm-up exercise that coordinates the breath, movement and energy flow images and works the muscles in the inner thighs, calves, ankles and feet.

Preparation

* Stand with one side of your body at arm's length away from a wall. Extend your arm out and place your fingertips or palm lightly on the wall for support. Check that you are standing upright and are not leaning into the wall.

* Keeping your heels together, turn your feet out to about 45 degrees. Make sure the whole of each foot is in contact with the floor and that your weight is evenly distributed over both feet. Aim to have your legs touching, from the heels right up to the top of the thighs, and gently press your legs together. As you bend and straighten the legs in this exercise, imagine your spine as a central pole that you slide up and down on without shifting your weight forwards or back.

* Breathe for a moment using the image of the Energy Fountain (see page 13), drawing the breath and energy in through the soles of your feet and sending the energy strongly up the backs of your legs. Visualize this powerful energy flow lifting you in the centre of your body and then escaping out through the crown of your head. See it cascading down and around the body so that your face, shoulders, ribs and arms are released into the downward flow back into the earth.

* Raise your free arm out to the side at shoulder height. Breathe in, elongating the spine and neck and lifting tall out of your hips, and go straight into the Half Knee Bends.

Half Knee Bends

* Breathe out firmly and bend your knees as deeply as you can, keeping the whole of each foot in contact with the floor. Resist the bending of the knees by imagining that you are pressing a wall on either side of you away with your knees. Keep the feet relaxed on the floor and release any gripping in the toes. Send energy out through your raised arms to help your balance (fig. right).

* Breathe in and start to slowly straighten your legs. Resist the straightening by imagining you are pressing a pillow between your legs as you straighten them. Hold on to this image until your legs are touching and pressing gently together. Keep reaching out through your free arm towards the far wall.

* Breathe out and slowly rise up onto half foot, raising the heels as far as is comfortable so that your weight is shifted onto your toes. Keep gently pressing your legs towards each other. Send the 'out' breath firmly down through the body and out through the feet, deep into the earth to form strong roots. At the same time, send energy out through your arms to the side walls to help you balance.

* Breathe in, drawing the breath up through your body and slowly lower your

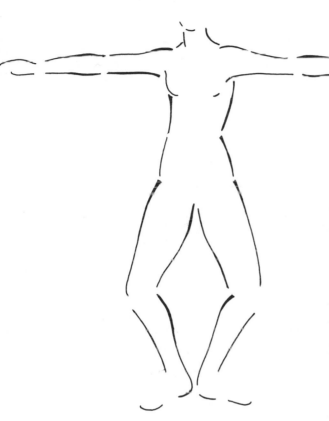

free arm up to the side at shoulder height and send energy out through the arms to the sides of the room. Bend as deeply as you can, keeping your heels on the floor, then raise the heels a little so that you continue the slow knee bend and go as deep as you can. Try not to collapse and just sit at the bottom of the knee bend but keep the movement controlled. As you bend your knees, your supporting hand should move down the wall with you so that it remains more or less at shoulder height (fig.overleaf).

* Breathe in and slowly straighten the legs, using the 'in' breath to fill and raise the body. Press that imaginary pillow between your legs as you straighten them. Replace your heels on the floor as soon as you can and then continue to slowly straighten the legs until they are touching. Keep both arms at shoulder height.

* Breathe out and rise onto half foot, gently pressing your legs together and sending the breath out firmly through your feet into the earth to form roots. Also send energy out through both arms to the sides of the room to balance you.

* Breathe in and slowly lower the heels as before, resisting the lowering by elongating through the spine. Bring your free arm down by your side.

* Turn around and use the other arm for support on the wall and begin again with the Half Knee Bends.

* Try the whole exercise twice through in total. Then shake out any tension in the arms and legs.

heels to the floor. Resist the lowering of the heels by focusing on the upward flow of energy that is lifting your upper body. Imagine the lowering of the heels as an elongation of the legs away from the upper body.

* Repeat the whole sequence once more, then go straight into the Full Knee Bends.

Full Knee Bends

* Breathe out and bend your knees, pushing away an imaginary wall to the left and right of you with your knees. Keep your

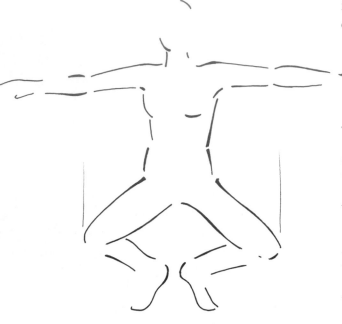

you, you can begin to add the energy flow images. All the sensations will eventually come together.

*13 BOUNCE AND LEG STRETCH

An energetic warm-up exercise for the legs.

Preparation

* Stand in the centre of your exercise space, with your feet as wide apart as your hips.
* Curl your head over towards your chest then curl your spine forwards as far as is comfortable. Let the spine, shoulders and arms hang down for a moment. As you breathe out, elongate and release the spine.

Sequence

* Bounce down to the floor into a crouching position, bending the knees and taking your heels off the floor. Place the palms of your hands in front of you on the floor. From this crouching position, bounce the hips up and down five or six times. As you bounce, move from crouching with the heels off the floor to semi-straightened legs with the heels on the floor (fig. right). Finish back in the crouching position.
* Over a count of five or six place the heels on the floor and slowly straighten your legs in one smooth movement. Aim to leave your hands, chest and head where they are

Notes

* The individual movements involved in this exercise are really quite simple but they become most effective when you incorporate all the ideas of resistance and energy flow. The idea of resisting something imaginary is very powerful, so be careful at first. Begin by creating the resistance images – the walls, the pillow and the elongation of the spine to lower the heels. Work with just a little resistance at first and then gradually increase it.
* There are several layers to this exercise and many things to try and hold in your Mind's Eye at once. When you have the resistance images clearly in your mind, start to coordinate the movements with the 'in' and 'out' breaths. Later, when the breathing and the images of resistance are familiar to

and lift only the hips. Breathe out along the spine and through the crown of the head, elongating the spine, then repeat the bounces and the stretch.

* Repeat the bounces and the stretch about five times in total.

*14 DRAWING ENERGY

A revitalizing and renewing exercise which draws life energy in and forcefully expels the old and the used

Preparation

* Sit on the floor on your mat or towel, with the soles of your feet together. Let your knees drop outwards towards the floor. Have your feet as close to your body as feels comfortable, as long as the base of your spine is straight and upright. If your feet do not meet when your spine is upright, place the soles about 12 inches (30 cm) apart, still facing each other, and drop the knees outwards.

Sequence

* Begin by breathing in and elongating the spine. Use the breath to lift your body up out of the hips and legs. Continue to breathe and try to maintain this lift. Raise both arms out in front at shoulder height to prepare.

* Using a rowing motion, on a strong 'in' breath, pull your arms towards your chest as if drawing life energy into your body. Without moving your feet, curve your pelvis and allow your spine to curve and rock backwards as far as it can (fig. overleaf top). Lift your bent arms up and circle them towards your ears in preparation for the next movement.

* With the 'out' breath, lift up through your spine and throw your arms out in front of you, as if casting off the breath and

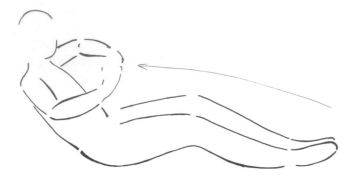

old energy. Let your body stretch forwards with the momentum of the throw. Really push the breath out as if trying to rid yourself of toxins, sending them out through your arms and fingers, through the top of your head and firmly out through your mouth. Make the breath audible as you send it out, emptying the lungs completely (fig. right)

* Breathe in and draw the arms towards your chest again to repeat the exercise.

* Repeat about ten times.

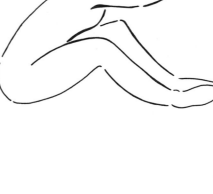

Notes

* The two motions – drawing back and curving the spine with the 'in' breath, and rising up and throwing the body forwards with the 'out' breath – together form a circle. Try to develop a confident, continuous rhythm to the circle.

* This exercise may make you a little light-headed at first with so much energy and breath being shifted through the body. If this is the case, return to centre, sitting with a straight spine, and breathe gently for a few moments before getting up or continuing the exercise.

STEP 2

UPPER BODY

1 TOXIN RELEASE

This exercise releases the powerful muscles that support the head and attach it to the shoulders. These muscles often hold a large amount of tension, thus storing waste and toxins.

Preparation

* Stand tall with your feet as wide apart as your hips and take a moment to breathe.

Sequence

* Breathe in and extend the left arm out to the side slightly. Deliberately send energy down through that hand into the floor to form a strong connection.
* Breathe out and tilt your head gently over to the right side, keeping the neck long. Take care not to crunch the head down towards your right shoulder. Keep facing front and reach with the top of your head towards the top of the right-hand wall and ceiling. With the left arm, send energy down towards the bottom of the left-hand wall and floor. Be aware that you are making a strong diagonal line from the top of the head to the fingertips of your left hand and beyond. Relax the chin and the jaw.
* Stay in that position and breathe in, drawing air into the tension in the neck. Imagine you are expanding and releasing the muscles with the breath.
* Make a controlled, drawn-out 'out' breath and send the air out both through the top of the head and also down through the arm and fingers. Release a little in the direction of the stretch. Imagine that as you

are stretched in two directions, you are creating a clear space in the neck and shoulder.
* Each time you breathe in, imagine you are drawing the breath directly into the space you have created. Allow the breath to dissipate the tension, leaving the neck and shoulder muscles malleable and free. On each 'out' breath send the waste and toxins strongly out of your body through the top of your head and down through the fingers.
* Repeat the stretch about three times on this side.
* To come out of the stretch, slowly roll your head down to the right side then forwards towards your chest. Use an 'in' breath to inflate the upper back and uncurl to the upright position.
* Now repeat the stretch with the head to the left and the arm reaching away to the right (fig. right).
* Try the whole exercise twice to the right and twice to the left, alternating sides. Roll the head forwards each time to change from one side to another. Try eventually to get a rhythm going with the breath.

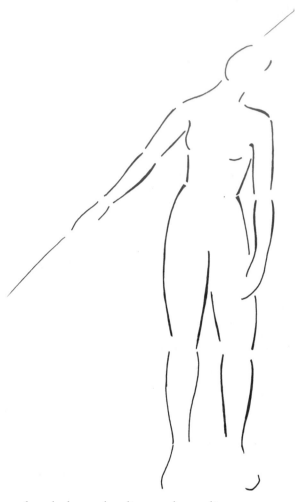

Toxin Release Variation

* Go into the exercise as before. In this variation you are going to do a stronger stretch on each 'out' breath.
* Once in the stretch, breathe in and raise your head about an inch (2.5 cm). Bring your extended arm down towards the side of your body then, curving your arm, take the hand up the side of your body as if gathering the air into your side.
* On the 'out' breath, elongate the neck and head along the diagonal, sending energy up through the crown of your head. At the same time, send the arm strongly out and down on the diagonal as if shooting the gathered air out and away through the fingertips.
* Repeat about three or four times.
* To come out of the stretch, roll your head forwards as before and slowly uncurl to the upright position.
* Repeat on the left side, then repeat on more on each side, alternating sides.

Notes

* The arm should draw continuous, uninterrupted circles throughout the breathing. Try to find a firm rhythm for the arm movement and the strong 'out' breath. This variation should be more energized than the original exercise.

2 SIDE STRETCH

A deep stretch for the shoulders, neck, torso, waist and hips.

Preparation

* Stand with your feet as wide apart as your hips and unlock the back of the knees.
* Take a moment to pass your Mind's Eye through your body to check that you are not gripping or holding muscles unnecessarily. If you are, release them with an 'out' breath.

Sequence

* Breathe in and lift one arm, drawing an arc from your side to above your head and reaching as far away from the body as you can. Leave the other arm relaxed by your side (fig. right).

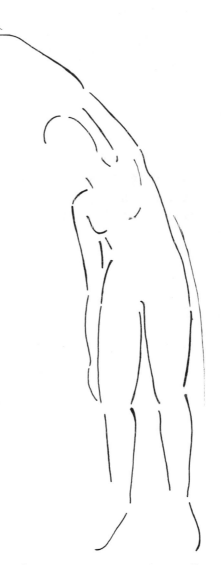

* On the 'out' breath, reach diagonally up over your head to the top of the opposite wall. Take four or five small bounces over into the stretch, and let your body curve over as far as it can. Try not to collapse in the waist, but continue reaching up and out, keeping the waist long on both sides. Stay in the stretch.
* On the next 'in' breath, do a further four or five small bounces. Imagine the breath and the energy entering through your out-

stretched fingertips and also up through your feet. Let the air expand your torso, creating space in the muscles and elongating your body.

* With the 'out' breath, come out of the stretch by rolling your upper body and arm forwards until you are curved over both legs equally.

* With the next 'in' breath, fill the spine from the base upwards and uncurl to the upright position.

* Breathe out and consciously release any 'held' muscles and unlock the knees. You are ready to repeat the exercise to the other side on the next 'in' breath.

* Try this twice on each side, alternating sides.

Notes

* The whole cycle takes six breaths to each side: 'in' as you raise your arm, 'out' for four or five bounces, 'in' for a further four or five bounces, 'out' as you release the stretch and curve over, 'in' to uncurl the spine, and 'out' to release. Try to maintain a slow but steady rhythm to the breathing.

* As you stretch, try taking your Mind's Eye into the side of your body and actually visualize the muscles opening and relinquishing tension. Send the breath out firmly through the fingers and down through the legs and feet, allowing it to clear the toxins and stiffness along the way.

* You will feel the stretch first of all in the opening of the shoulder joint and in the ribs and probably also in the upper arm. Later, as you become more flexible you will feel the stretch in the waist and in the powerful hip and bottom muscles which extend into the lower back.

* This exercise can be done without the bounces, using a more powerful still method of stretching, breathing into the stretch and releasing further with the 'out' breath.

Side Stretch Variation

* To extend the stretch into the the hips and bottom, start as before, making sure your legs are straight but not locked.

* As you reach up and over into the stretch, bend your knees, keeping the whole of each foot in contact with the floor. Take care to keep the spine in the vertical plane – don't tilt it forwards or back – and keep the hips facing front. This time as you bounce with the 'out' and 'in' breaths you will feel a deeper stretch that reaches into the lower back.

* To come out of this deeper stretch, it is important to roll your upper body and curve forwards over your bent legs. Then, with the final 'in' breath, draw the breath in through the soles of your feet and slowly straighten your legs while uncurling the spine.

3 CONCENTRIC CIRCLES

This exercise opens and works the shoulder joint and opens the chest. It is made up of three different circling movements that gradually increase in size. Any one of these circling movements can be used on its own to work the upper body if you prefer.

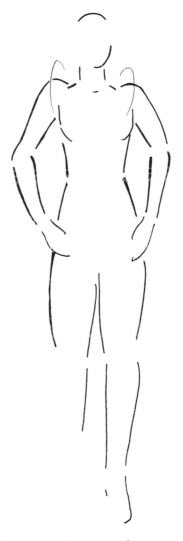

Preparation

* Stand with your feet as wide apart as your hips. Let your shoulders relax and drop away from the neck, and release any other muscles that are held tense in the body. Relax your arms and let them hang down by your sides. Breathe.

Circle one

* You are going to move your shoulders in a backward circle. Start by lifting them up towards your ears as far as they will go. Continue the circle by taking your shoulders backwards behind you. This movement will open the chest and bring your shoulder blades closer together. Continue the circle by taking your shoulders down as far away from your neck and head as possible, then bring them to the front as if to meet each other. Carry on up towards your ears again in a smooth circle (fig. right). Try four rotations.

* Now reverse the direction. Circle your shoulders up towards your ears, then forwards and down as if to meet each other. Continue by taking them down away from your head and neck, then up and back, opening the chest and bringing the shoulder blades closer together. Do four rotations, keeping the movement as smooth as possible and without tension. Make the circles as large as possible, keeping your shoulders very open. Breathe naturally and keep the rise and fall of the chest relaxed.

* Repeat the backward and forward circles once more, doing four rotations of each, then flow smoothly into the second circling movement.

Circle two

* Bend your arms, bring your fingers up and place them on your shoulders. You are going to use the points of your elbows to draw a backward circle in the air. Bring the elbows up together in front of your face. Lift them over your head, keeping them as close together as possible. Open the elbows wide as you circle down behind your body, and then continue down and forwards so that the elbows meet each other. Again, do four smooth circles, ending with the elbows together up above your head (fig. left).

* Now circle the elbows forwards in front of your face and then down by the sides of the body, up and back behind you, bringing them close together as soon as possible to finish above your head. This movement will feel a little like the butterfly swimming stroke. Continue for four rotations, keeping the circles as large as possible and without tension.

* Repeat the backward and forward circles with the elbows again, then flow smoothly into the third circling movement.

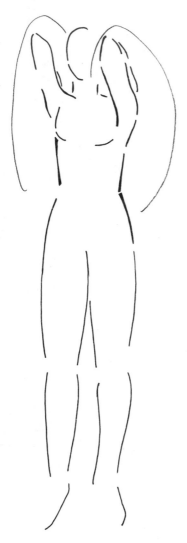

Circle three

* The elbows will now be up above your head after the last forward elbow circle. Uncurl and extend the arms above your head and then begin to circle your straight arms backwards. Circle gently, taking care not to lock the elbows. Draw a large circle with the tips of your fingers. Imagine your fingers are tracing circles of light in the air. Do four rotations and finish as your arms come up in front of your chest and up over your head.

* Smoothly reverse the direction to circle the arms forwards. Again, do four rotations and finish with your arms over your head.

* Repeat the backward and forward circles with straight arms once more.

Notes

* Proceed very gently at first with this exercise, since your shoulder joints and chest may not be accustomed to so much movement. You may find that you tend to overcompensate for a lack of shoulder mobility by moving your head forwards and back. Try to hold the head tall throughout with a long, relaxed neck, and keep your spine fluid and upright. Imagine the arms are drawing circles in the air independently from the rest of your body. Always pass the arms as close together as possible over the head. Imagine energy and breath filling the neck and flowing out through the crown of the head during the exercise.

* You may also experience what some people have described as 'gravel' in the shoulder, which is not painful but sounds loud. This is the sound of the joint working beyond its accustomed range of motion and is nothing to worry about. The joint will lubricate itself over a matter of weeks or months and this effect should disappear, although it might return if you take a break from exercising.

* Once you become familiar with the directions and patterns of the movements, focus on the circling movement travelling through your energy field. Be aware of how you affect the energy in your field as the size of the circles increases in the three different circling movements. Notice how much more energy flows through the body as you draw larger and larger circles away from your body with your shoulders, elbows and then the fingers.

Concentric Circles Variation

* Do all the backward circles of circles one, two and three. Do four rotations of each, making them flow non-stop into each other. Then reverse the direction and do all the forward circles. Aim to make the transitions between the steps fluid so that the circling is uninterrupted. Try this variation twice through.

4 ELBOW PRESS

A gentle exercise that strengthens and stretches the shoulders and tones the backs of the chest and the upper arms.

Preparation

* Stand in the centre of your exercise space with your feet as wide apart as your hips and relaxed on the floor. Reach your arms out wide to the side into the Open Star position (see page 13). Breathe for a moment in this position, lengthening the arms and opening your chest and back.

Sequence

* Keeping your arms reaching out, bring them forwards at shoulder height to meet each other in front of your chest. As they come close, bend your elbows so that your hands are above your head, with palms facing you and elbows directly in front of your chest. Hold the arms about three inches (7.5 cm) apart. Imagine there is a pillow or

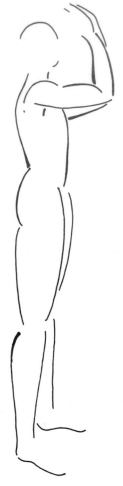

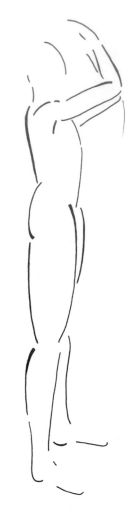

cushion between your arms and that you are pressing into this to hold it in place (fig. above).

* Keep the forearms parallel and, with an 'out' breath, press them into the pillow towards each other for a count of eight.

* Breathe in, release the press and relax for a moment, then repeat the press about four times, pressing into the pillow with the 'out' breath and releasing and relaxing with the 'in' breath.

* Now breathe out, pressing the forearms into the pillow and at the same time lift your elbows upwards. Keep the forearms parallel. Press in and upwards for a count of eight as you breathe out and hold on to the pillow throughout (fig.above). Your arms will not lift very high – about one or two inches (2.5–5 cm).

* Breathe in and release the press, lowering your elbows back to chest height, then breathe out and repeat the press and lift for another count of eight. Keep the arms parallel throughout the press, and don't allow them to touch. Try this about four times in total.

* Now repeat the whole exercise once more, making the movements continuous and fluid. Keep your breathing soft, and release any tension in the neck and jaw.

* To finish, breathe in and release the press. Lower the elbows to chest height and straighten your arms out in front. Send energy out through the arms as you carry them out to the sides, reaching away from the body, to finish in the Open Star position.

5 HAND AND ARM CIRCLES

This exercise works the wrists, elbow and shoulder joints and improves their mobility.

Preparation

* Stand in the centre of your exercise space, with your feet as wide apart as your hips, and raise your arms in front of you to about waist height. Imagine your arms are placed on a surface of water. Let them float there, supported by the water, without any effort. Allow the arms to bend naturally at the elbows, and release your shoulders.

Sequence

* Flex the hands down at the wrist and begin to circle the hands inwards, circling from the wrists. Take the hands out to the sides, then up and inwards to meet each

other. Do four circles.

* Relax the hands and flex the forearms down from the elbow. Start to circle the forearms inwards, circling from the elbows. Circle the forearms out to the sides, then up and in to meet each other and continue for four circles. Try to keep the upper arms still as you do this – imagine they are still supported by the water (fig. below).

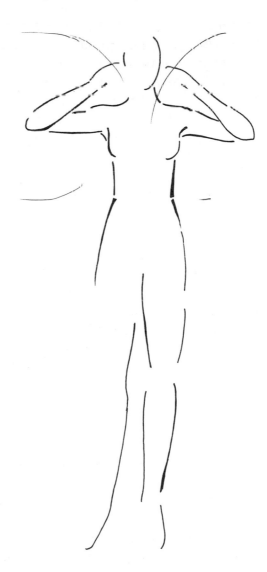

* Relax the forearms, and start to circle the whole of each arm from the shoulder. Keep the arms relaxed and slightly bent. Take them down, out to the sides, up and then let them cross in front of you. Continue for four circles and finish in the starting position with arms extended in front at waist height.

* Let the arms rest on the water and release any tension. Now begin the sequence again, this time circling outwards. Flex the hands down, circle the hands towards each other, then up and out to the sides. Continue for four circles. Next, do four outward circles from the elbows, keeping the upper arms still. Now, using the whole of the arms from the shoulders, do four outward circles with arms relaxed. Shake out the arms to finish.

* Repeat the whole exercise again.

Notes

* As you become familiar with the directions and the sensations of isolating different parts of your arm, try to make the transitions flow one into another so that the whole exercise is one continuous movement. Consciously relax the shoulders throughout the exercise.

Hand and Arm Circles Variation

* This is a little like a tongue-twister. Begin with the inward circles with the hands. Once you have established those, add the inward forearm circles while maintaining the hand circles. Finally, begin to circle inwards from the shoulder using the whole arm, while maintaining the other two circling movements.

* Now begin with outward hand circles and gradually add the other two. It's not important to be able to do all of them at once, but it's an interesting exercise for testing coordination!

6 WINGS

This exercise encourages mobility in the shoulder joints and strengthens the arms. The exercise uses the rise and fall of the breath as the impetus for the arm movement. The arms echo the movement of the breath.

Preparation

* Stand in the centre of your exercise space, with your feet as wide apart as your hips and your arms hanging relaxed by your sides.

* Pass your Mind's Eye through your body and release any holding in the muscles. Release the throat and chest and the hip and thigh muscles. Take a deep breath in, filling the lungs right down to the stomach, and then control the release of the breath out. Empty the lungs totally and for a moment be without breath before replenishing the body. Take about five full and controlled breaths and establish a calm, steady rhythm, then begin.

Sequence

* With a deep 'in' breath, use the image of the incoming breath to raise your arms to the sides. As you lift your arms, lead with the elbows, tips of the elbows pointing upwards. Allow the forearms and hands to hang down naturally from the elbows. Imagine that the air is billowing and filling the space under your arms and lifting them. Lift as high as is comfortable for the shoulder joints (fig. below).

* Now turn the arms so that the tips of the elbows are pointing to the floor. Keep the same angle in the arms so that the forearms and hands are now pointing upwards. With the 'out' breath, press down with the elbows and the backs of your arms, as if pushing away a huge body of air (fig. below). Use the same image to control the breath out of the lungs and empty them completely. Direct the elbows into the sides of the body at the waist and finish with the elbows and the backs of the arms touching your sides.

* Breathe in and replenish the body with air. Let the air fill and lift the space under the arms, raising them from the elbows, and continue as before.

* Try four or six repetitions in total. On the 'in' breath, allow the body to be guided by the breath so that the movement flows with it, and then on the 'out' breath consciously press the air and breath away.

Wings Variation

This variation helps develop coordination in the upper body.

* Start by stretching the arms out to the sides at shoulder height. Breathe, opening the chest and the shoulders wide to the sides.

* As you breathe in, raise the right arm up by the elbow as before, but this time turn the left arm over and press down with the elbow into the waist, taking the whole slow 'in' breath to complete the movement.

* Breathe out and press down into the waist with the right elbow and at the same time lift the left elbow. Continue alternating arms and try eight to ten repetitions.

Notes

* This movement will feel completely different from the original, like a wave passing from side to side through the upper body, from the right fingertips through to the left fingertips and back again. Once you are comfortable with the coordination of the movement, focus on making the wave pass fluidly and continuously from one hand to the other.

*7 ARM PRESS

A strengthening and stretching exercise for the shoulders, chest and backs of the arms. The muscles in the back of the shoulder and the back of the upper arm are often difficult to isolate.

Preparation

* Stand in the centre of your exercise space with your feet as wide apart as your hips. Lift both arms in front of you to shoulder height, with the palms of the hands facing each other.

Sequence

* Breathe in and open your arms out wide to the sides. Turn the arms so that the palms are facing the floor, and carry the arms on to finish directly behind you with palms facing each other. As you move the arms, reach out a long way from the body. The arms will lower naturally as they move behind the body, but try to keep them as high as you can.

* Breathe out over a count of ten and gently press the palms and fingertips towards each other, keeping the arms as high as you can. At the same time, curve your head and upper spine over a little towards your chest

and bend the knees slightly (fig. below).
* After the count of ten, breathe in and uncurl the spine to upright and straighten your legs. Release the press but leave the arms in place behind you.
* Breathe out over a count of ten, again

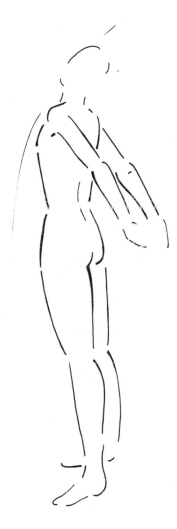

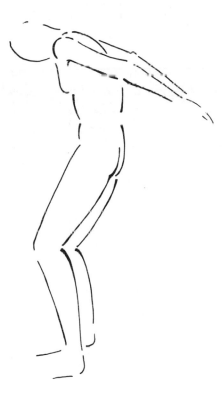

pressing the fingertips and palms towards each other. This time open the chest a little to the ceiling, inclining the head back as a natural extension of the spine (fig. right).
* After the count of ten, breathe in, straighten the spine and release the press, leaving the arms where they are.
* Continue alternating the press with bent knees and curved spine, with the press with straight legs and chest open to the ceiling. With each 'in' breath release the press and

relax a little. Try ten lots of presses in total.
* To finish, do not drop the arms in relief immediately behind you. Breathe in and release the arms from the last ten-count press. Lift the head and spine to upright, and very slowly carry the arms out to the sides at shoulder level, reaching out a long way from the body. Carry them on in front of you and then slowly lower them to your sides. Shake out any tension in the shoulders and arms.

Notes

* If the curving or opening of the spine feels awkward as you press, the arm press can equally be done without them. Go into the exercise exactly as before, but hold the spine upright throughout the exercise and keep the knees slightly bent. Follow the breathing, counting and release as described for the original exercise.

*8 FLAMENCO CONTRACT AND OPEN

A beautiful movement that opens the chest and back and increases the mobility in the upper body. It imitates the movement used in Flamenco dance.

Preparation

* Stand in the centre of your exercise space, with your feet as wide apart as your hips and arms relaxed by your sides.
* Breathe and release the shoulders and chest. Breathe in and bend your legs, keeping your heels on the floor. Use the breath to lengthen the spine. Stay tall and upright.

Sequence

* Breathe out for a count of four or five. As you breathe out, draw the backs of the hands in a large arc in front of you so that they meet and then cross in front of you. Imagine you are pressing the backs of the

hands through water that is all around you, and feel the resistance given by the water. At the same time, curve your upper body, chest and head over towards the hands (fig. below). Imagine that the line of your spine and the back of your head to where the hands meet form one continuous curve.
* As you breathe in, lift your arms swiftly and gather the body up to the upright position but keep your knees bent. Still using the 'in' breath, open the arms above your head, leading with the elbows. Slowly draw the elbows down behind your back towards each other, as if they could meet. Open the chest and upper body to the ceiling, letting your head lean back as a natural extension

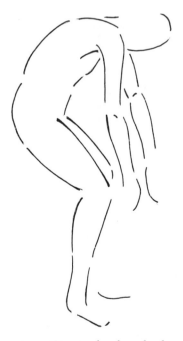

of the spine. Carry the head, do not let it just drop back (fig. right).
* Breathe out over four or five counts and begin the curving movement from this

arched position. Start by drawing the backs of the hands towards each other, arcing them around in front of you, as if moving through water. Let the body follow this movement, curving forwards in the chest and shoulders, then allow the head and spine to complete the curve over.

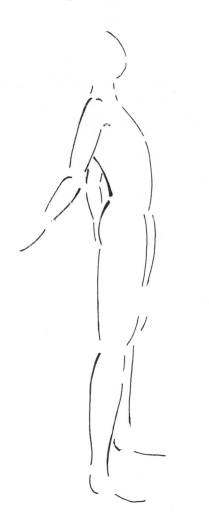

* Try about ten careful forward and back movements and then shake out the arms, shoulders and upper body. Aim for the whole exercise to flow, one movement into

another, and yet let the movements have strength.

*9 TOWEL STRETCH

An effective stretch for the shoulders, arms, chest and waist.

Preparation

* Take a hand towel or large tea towel and gather it up so that it forms a long, thin oblong. Take one end of the towel in each hand. Hold the towel taut between your hands in a light fist, as if holding the handlebars of a bicycle. As this is a strenuous exercise for the shoulder joints, begin very gently. The closer together your hands, the harder the exercise, so start off with your hands at least three feet (90 cm) apart and at the very ends of the towel. Over the next few months, as your shoulder joints become more mobile, aim to gradually reduce the distance between your hands.
* Place your arms down by your sides so that the towel lies across your thighs. Breathe, and let your shoulders drop away from your neck. Keep the towel taut between your two hands and keep your arms straight throughout the exercise, but take care not to lock your elbows or hold the arms rigid. Try to maintain an energy flow out through the arms so that they feel fluid yet strong.

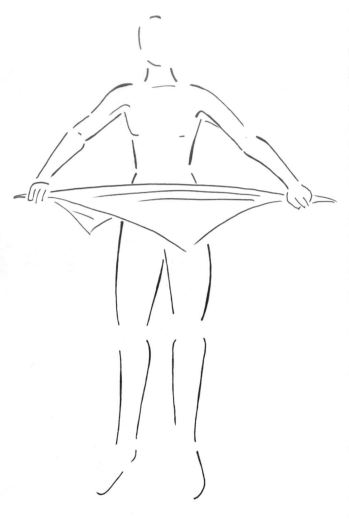

* Breathe out and repeat the bounces.
* Repeat the bounces about three times in total, then lower the arms to the starting position across the front of the thighs.
* Now breathe in and raise the arms straight up in front of you until the towel is directly over your head. Breathe out and slowly lower the towel down behind your body until it touches the backs of your thighs.
* Breathe in and slowly raise the towel until it is directly over your head. This is a strenuous movement, so release the towel if you need to, then take it up again above your head. Eventually try to perform this movement holding onto the towel throughout.
* Breathe out and slowly lower the towel to the starting position.
* Try this whole pattern three or four times in total.

Sequence

* Breathe in and raise the arms straight up in front of you (fig. above) until the towel is directly over your head.
* Breathe out for six counts and at the same time gently bounce the towel backwards just behind your head, opening the shoulders.
* Breathe in and bring your arms forwards again to just above your head. Release the shoulders and elongate the spine and the neck.

Towel Stretch Variation

* Do the exercise as before and finish by holding the towel taut between both hands and directly above your head.
* Relax your shoulders and check that there is energy flowing through your arms and that the elbows are not locked. You are going to draw a circle with the upper body, all the while holding the towel with outstretched arms. Keep the towel above your head the whole time and keep your head in the centre of your raised arms.
* Breathe out and lean over to the right side (fig. right). Continue the circle by bending your knees and curving your spine over forwards until your outstretched arms are

directly in front of you and your upper body is curved over your legs.

* Breathe in and continue the circle up to the left side, reaching out with the arms. As you come up to the side, turn the upper body as soon as you can so that you are

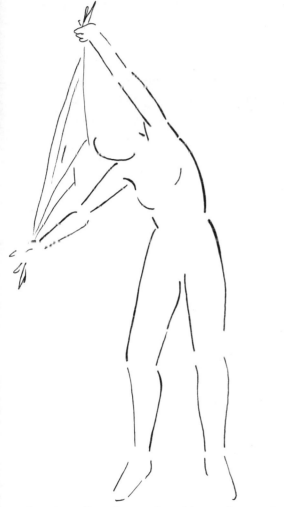

leaning directly to the side and your body and head is facing front. Straighten your legs as you raise up to the centre to finish with the towel above your head.

* Continue as above until you have completed four circles to the right. Then reverse

the direction of the circle by breathing out as you lean to the left side, then bending your legs and curving your spine over your bent legs. With the 'in' breath, lift up to the right and back to centre. Complete four circles to the left.

* To finish, lower the arms gently down in front of you. Release one end of the towel and shake out your arms and shoulders.

Notes

* This is a strenuous exercise and should be performed with care. Control the movement of the upper body and arms at all times. Do not let them swing with their own weight, as any extra force or impetus may cause injury.

*10 SHOULDER CHAIR STRETCH

This stretch opens the chest and shoulders and elongates the spine. You will need a chair for this exercise. The higher the chair back, the easier the stretch. The lower the chair back, the greater the stretch for the spine.

Preparation

*Stand behind the chair and place your hands lightly on the chair back so that they are shoulder-width apart.

71

Sequence

* Breathe out, curling your head down towards the top of the chair and curving your spine. Then take two or three small steps backwards away from the chair until your spine and arms are straightened and your legs are directly under your hips (fig. below).

* Breathe through your spine for a moment, keeping your spine long and straight. Do not allow it to sink down between your shoulders towards the floor. Hold your head straight between your arms as a natural extension of your spine.

* Breathe out and, leaving the hands where they are, bend your knees as deeply as you can. Keep the arms and spine long and let them move as one. Send the breath out through the top of your head and out through the arms and hands into the chair and also, if you can visualize it, send it down through the legs into the floor, elongating the spine.

* Draw the breath in and slowly inflate and straighten the legs. Check that your spine, arms and head make one long, straight line.

* Repeat the deep bend on the 'out' breath and, on the 'in' breath, inflate and straighten the legs. Feel as if the legs are mirroring the movement of the breath.

* Breathe out, curl your pelvis and curve your spine. Start to walk towards the chair, curling your head towards your chest.

* Breathe in as you arrive at the chair and uncurl to the upright position.

* Breathe out and relax before repeating the exercise. Do the whole exercise at least four times.

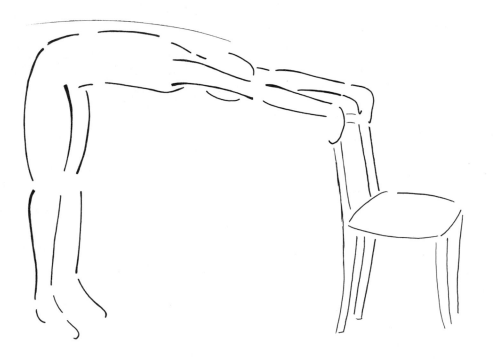

STEP 3

LOWER BODY

1 FOOT STRENGTHENER

A very simple exercise to strengthen the arches of the feet.

Preparation
* Stand with your feet as wide apart as your hips. Spread your feet on the floor. Keep the toes long and without tension, and feel the whole of each foot in contact with the floor. With an 'out' breath release any tension in the upper body.

Sequence
* You are going to work one foot at a time. Keeping the toes long, press them into the floor and while drawing the arch of the foot up towards you as far as you can (fig. right). The toes will eventually lift off the floor.

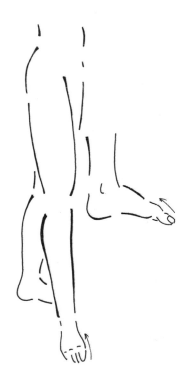

* Lift the toes and arch of the foot completely off the floor, flexing the foot so that the weight rests on the ball of the heel. Stretch the toes forwards, away from the heel, to elongate the foot, then place the toes back on the floor.
* Repeat the exercise with the other foot. Do 20 in total with alternate feet.

Notes
* Once you have the sensation of the movement and can repeat it with ease, focus on a point at eye level in front of you rather than down at your feet.
* Breathe naturally and let energy travel throughout the whole body. Aim to move smoothly from one foot to the other.

2 FLEX AND PUSH

This exercise strengthens the thighs, calves, ankles and feet and helps develop your sense of balance.

Preparation
* Stand in the centre of your exercise space, with your feet parallel and as wide apart as your hips.
* Place your arms wide to the sides at shoulder height, just forward of the body line and within eyesight. Throughout the exercise, send energy out through the arms and fingers to the walls on either side of you. This creates a two-way pull which,

together with the opening of the chest, will help you keep your balance during the exercise.
* Find a point or object at eye level in front of you that you can focus on. If you concentrate the eyes on this point during the exercise this will also help with your balance.

Sequence
* Breathe in and brush your right leg forwards away from you, pressing the foot into the floor as you brush it forwards until

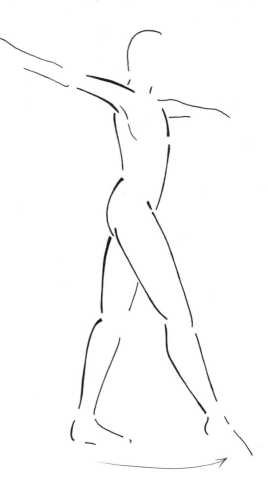

it comes just off the floor in front of you. Keep the energy reaching a long way beyond the body through the right leg and toes. All of the weight of the body is now supported on the left leg (fig.left).

* Breathe out and drop all your weight forwards onto your right leg, bending the right knee deeply.

* Breathe in and flex the toes of the right foot back towards you, rocking your weight onto the right heel and straightening the right leg. As you do this, some of your weight will shift back onto the left leg. Send energy down the back of the right leg and through the heel into the floor. You should feel a stretch in the back of the right calf (fig.right).

* Breathe out and shift your weight forwards again onto the right foot, bending the knee deeply as before.

* Breathe in and push off the floor with the right leg, so that the weight of the body shifts to the left foot. Leave the right foot extended and raised just off the floor in front of you. Imagine your leg is very long and extends beyond the ends of the toes.

* With the 'out' breath, brush the right foot back towards you, pressing into the floor as you draw the foot back under the body to finish in the starting position with your weight evenly distributed on both feet.

* Repeat this whole sequence with the left foot.

* Now, do the exercise again, starting with the right foot, but this time brush the foot directly out to the side instead of in front, toes pointing forwards. Press into the floor until the foot lifts just off the floor.

* On the 'out' breath, drop your weight to the side onto the right foot, bending the right knee deeply.

* Breathe in, flexing the right foot and straightening the leg. The toes point to the front all the time. Some of your weight will transfer onto the supporting leg as you flex the foot. Send energy down the back of the right leg, through the heel and into the floor.

* Breathe out and shift the weight into a deep bend on the right leg again.

* Breathe in and push off the floor with your right leg, extending the leg just off the floor.

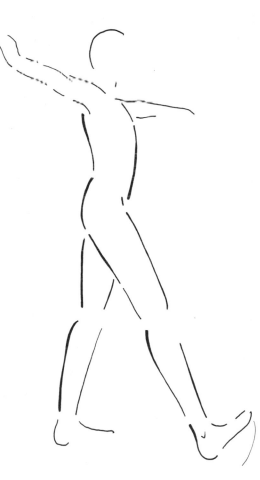

* Breathe out and draw the foot across the floor until it returns directly under the body and your weight is evenly distributed between both feet.
* Repeat to the left side.
* Try the whole exercise twice through in total, alternating legs: right leg, then left leg to the front, followed by right leg, then left leg to the side, and repeat.

Notes

* It is not necessary to lift the leg higher than one or two inches (2.5–5cm) off the floor.
* Strength is developed by pressing into the floor as you brush the working foot forwards or sideways. When the foot leaves the floor, continue to elongate the leg and foot and imagine that you are sending energy out of it and back into the floor, way in front or to the side of you. Try to work in a fluid way by joining all the movements together so that they work naturally with the breath.

3 LEG BRUSHES

A strengthening exercise for the whole of the legs, the feet and hips.

Preparation

* Stand next to a wall or support yourself using the back of a chair. Place your left hand lightly on the wall or on the back of the chair for balance and extend your right arm out at shoulder height, just in front of the line of the body. Stand with the heels touching and the toes turned out to about 45 degrees.

Sequence

* Brush your right leg out in the direction of the toes. Keep the leg straight and continue the brush until the foot is completely extended and only the tips of the toes are in contact with the floor.
* Slowly draw the foot back towards you, brushing through the floor until the heels meet again.
* Breathe in and brush the foot out again, this time brushing the foot more energetically so that it comes off the floor. Let the foot elongate as before so that the tips of the toes are the last thing to leave the floor. Continue lifting the leg up, using the momentum of the brush and the 'in' breath, then bend the knee so that the toes touch the inside of the supporting knee.
* Breathe out and lower the right foot to the floor. Keep the foot close to the supporting leg as you lower it all the way down. Finish with heels touching and toes turned out to 45 degrees so that you are ready to start again from the beginning.
* Try between six and ten of these brushing and circling movements, then turn around and place your right hand lightly on the wall or the chair for support and extend your left arm out at shoulder height. Now do six to ten brushes and circles working with the left leg (fig.right).

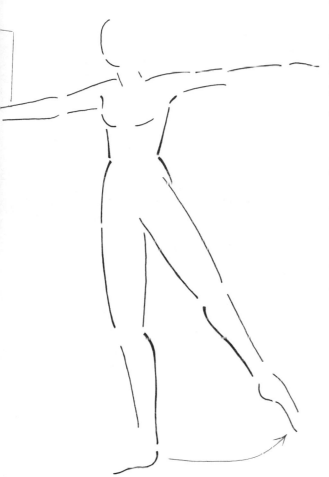

4 HEEL RAISERS

An exercise to strengthen and stretch the feet, ankles and calves and to improve balance. Heel Raisers uses a four-breath pattern of coordinated breathing that integrates the whole body into the exercise.

Preparation

* Stand facing a wall so that you are at arm's length away from the wall with your body square to it. Your feet are parallel and as wide apart as your hips, and your weight is centred over both feet. Release any gripping in your feet and in the fronts of the ankles.
* Place your fingertips or palms lightly on the wall for balance. Take a moment to breathe. Breathe in to start.

Four-breath cycle

* Breathe out and bend your knees deeply, keeping the whole of each foot in contact with the floor. Think of this movement as a relaxation as if you were simply folding the front of the ankles. Imagine sending the breath up through the spine, keeping the spine straight and long, and also down through the soles of the feet into the earth.
* With the 'in' breath, draw energy into the body through the soles of the feet and also through the crown of the head. As the breath fills the body, straighten your legs.
* Breathe out firmly and come up onto half foot by lifting your heels off the floor as high as you can, keeping your weight centred over the toes. Send the breath down

Notes

* Focus at first on the sensation of the foot pushing through the floor as it brushes. When you begin to feel some resistance as you brush through the floor, you will find that the leg lifts a little higher when it leaves the floor.

through your feet and into the earth. Imagine the downward breath and energy

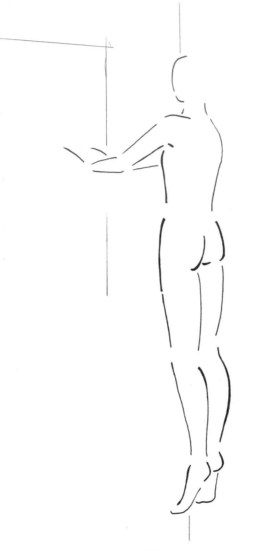

flow creating strong roots (fig. above).
* Breathe in, drawing breath and energy in through the soles of the feet and, at the same time, slowly lower the heels to the floor. Try to resist the lowering of the heels by focusing on the upward direction of the flowing energy. You should feel a two-way

pull as the body is drawn upwards with the breath and the legs are lengthened by the lowering of the heels. Feel as if you are growing. Hold on to this image until the whole foot is in contact with the floor.
* Repeat this sequence about eight times.

Notes

* To recap, the four breaths are: 'out' to bend the knees, 'in' to straighten the legs, 'out' to raise the heels and send down roots, 'in' to resist the lowering of the heels and elongate the body.
* Keep the rhythm of the breathing and the movement at a steady pace. There is a lot to concentrate on, so build up the layers slowly. Concentrate initially on familiarizing yourself with the mechanics of the exercise and the breathing. Once you are comfortable with these, then focus on the images and the direction of the energy. The image of casting energy firmly down as you rise up onto half foot creates a connection with the earth and gives you a strong sense of balance. Occasionally, practise taking your hands from the wall as you rise up and throw down energy. Feel as if you could balance there forever holding the image of roots beneath you.

Heel Raisers Variation

The movement pattern here is exactly the same as in the original exercise, but it is now flowing and coordinated with two breaths.

Two-breath cycle

* With an 'in' breath, draw energy into the body through the soles of the feet and bend the knees as deeply as you can, keeping the whole of each foot in contact with the floor.
* With the 'out' breath, strongly send the energy down through your whole body into the earth. Push up through the feet, straighten the legs and raise onto half foot. Be aware of the powerful line of energy running through the body, down the legs, through the toes and as far into the earth as you can imagine, forming your strong roots.
* With the 'in' breath, lower the heels, resisting the lowering as you draw energy in and up through the soles of the feet. When the whole foot is in contact with the floor, soften and bend the legs. Keep the image of an elongation and upward flow in the body as long as possible.
* Continue rising up onto half foot with each outward breath and lowering and bending with each inward breath. Connect the movements so that they become fluid and continuous.
* Try ten in total.

5 ZEN LEG LIFTS

This is a strenghtening exercise for the thigh muscles. They get their name because the whole focus of the exercise is on the outward flow of energy through the lifted leg and not on the muscular action or effort involved.

Preparation

* Stand with your left side at arm's length from a wall or supporting surface. Have your heels touching and toes slightly apart. Place your left hand lightly on the wall, with your arm outstretched. Stretch your right arm out to the side at shoulder height, slightly in front of the body, so that you are just aware of it out of the corner of your eye. Throughout the exercise your chest should feel open as you send energy out to the side through this arm. This will help to balance you. Release your shoulders and begin.

Sequence

* Breathe in and brush the right leg forwards. Keeping the leg straight, let it rise off the floor about six to twelve inches (15–30 cm). Imagine enormous amounts of energy or water coursing through the leg and out beyond the toes. Fix a point in front of you and direct the energy through the foot towards this point.
* Breathe out and bend the supporting leg. Stay very tall in the spine as you bend, and keep the energy flowing out to the same fixed point in front of you. Be aware that your right leg will raise naturally as you do this (fig. overleaf).
* Breathe in and slowly straighten the supporting leg, keeping the energy directed at the same fixed point in front of you. Imagine the energy in the legs is very fluid and fast-moving, even though your movements are slow. This will help the muscles to stay released and not go rigid.
* Keeping your right leg lifted, try this

* Breathe out and slowly bend the supporting leg. Focus on sending the energy strongly out to the same point, and maintain the image of the energy being fluid.

bending and straightening of the supporting leg four times.

* Breathe out and imagine that you are elongating the raised leg away from you. Slowly lower the leg, brushing it through the floor to join the left heel. If you feel any tension, shake out the legs and arms, then resume your starting position and continue.

* Now, breathe in and brush your right leg out to the side in the direction of the toes. Press into the floor as you brush, and then lift the leg off the floor as before. Send energy out through the leg and through the toes to a fixed point beyond you to the side.

* Without changing the point of focus of the energy, breathe in and straighten the supporting leg.

* Repeat the bending and straightening of the supporting leg four times, keeping the energy focus very powerful.

* Breathe out and elongate the right leg, then slowly lower it, brushing it through

the floor to join the left heel. Again, shake out your legs and arms if they are stiff and then resume the starting position.

* Now breathe in and brush the right leg directly behind you and lift it just off the floor. Send energy strongly out through the leg and toes to a point behind you.

* Breathe out and sink into the supporting leg. Feel the lifted leg rise a little as you continue to send energy out to the same point on the floor behind you (fig. near left).

* Breathe in and straighten the supporting leg. The lifted leg will lower a little so that it still directs energy to the same point. Do four lots of bending and straightening of the supporting leg.

* Breathe out and slowly lower the raised leg to the floor, sending energy out until the foot touches the floor. Brush the foot through the floor to join the left heel.

* Shake everything out and then turn around, place your right hand lightly on the wall for support and extend your left arm straight out at shoulder height for balance. Begin the whole exercise again with the left leg.

6 FRONT OF THIGH

This exercise elongates and opens the front of the body and the front of the hips, allowing a clear flow of energy. It also strengthens the backs of the thighs and the bottom.

Preparation

* Stand facing a wall at arm's length, with your body square to it. Reach your arms out in front at shoulder height and place your fingertips or palms lightly on the wall.

* Take a moment to breathe, lifting tall out of your hips, elongating your spine and neck and releasing any tension in your shoulders. Let your feet be soft on the floor.

Sequence

* Bend your right knee and lift your right foot up behind you towards your bottom. Take hold of your right ankle with your

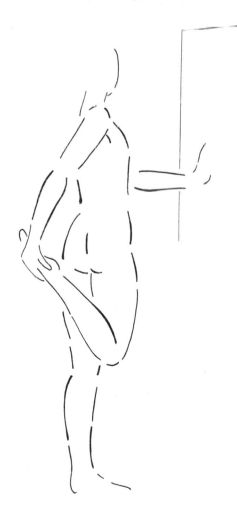

right hand. Keep the same alignment as if you were standing upright so that your right knee is next to your left knee. Release any tension. Drawing the breath through the body, gently pull your foot towards your bottom, feeling the elongation in the front of the right hip. Try not to sink into the left hip but stay lifted (fig. prev. page).

* Gently circle the right knee, doing five or six rotations in one direction and making the circles as large as is comfortable. Then reverse the direction and do five or six rotations in the other direction. Take the point where the knees are together as the front of the circle so that you circle slightly behind your body line. This will gently work the hip joint and open the front of the hip.

* Lift the right knee and arm slowly up behind you as far as is comfortable and hold for a count of ten. As you do so, tilt the body forwards a little so that you can lift the leg. Breathe in and out throughout the count of ten. Be aware of the circle created by your arm and lifted leg, and send energy through the circle – down the front of your body, through the thigh, circling into the hand, through the arm, opening the shoulder then back into the body. Breathe deliberately through this circle created by the right side of the body, but be aware of some breath as normal in the left side of the body (fig. right).

* Slowly lower the arm and knee, then release your hand and slowly place the right foot back on the floor. Breathe. Check that you are facing square to the wall, then repeat the whole sequence with the left leg.

* To finish, place both hands squarely on the wall in front of you at shoulder height.

Lift one foot up behind you so that the knee is lifted slightly behind the body line. Keeping it behind you, lift the knee and thigh in gentle bounces of one or two inches (2.5–5 cm) 10–20 times. Breathe throughout and keep the front and back of the body elongated and released. Imagine water or energy constantly flowing through the lifted thigh and escaping out through the lifted foot. Lower the leg and replace on the floor, then repeat the bounces with the other leg.

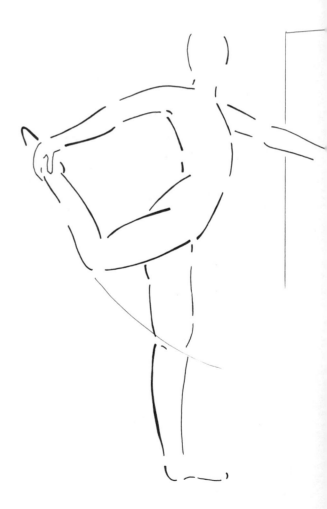

Front of Thigh Variation

Once you feel comfortable breathing and holding the arm and leg up in a circle as described above, you can increase its effectiveness by adding an isometric image.

* When you lift the leg and arm to form the circle, press the foot into the hand, as if your intention was to straighten the leg. At the same time, maintain your hold of the ankle and allow the body to tilt forwards towards the wall if necessary to enable this movement. Keep the breath moving around the circle made by the lifted leg and arm. Try to keep the whole action fluid by imagining the breath as coursing water running through the body, around the circle and back out again into the floor through the supporting foot and also out through the top of the head. You will find that the leg does not actually move, although the amount of energy passing through the movement will increase.
* To come out of this, release the isometric image and the energy images. Slowly lower the leg, still holding the ankle, then release your hand and place the foot on the floor.
* Repeat with the other leg.

7 FLEX AND STRETCH

A stretch for the legs, calves and feet.

Preparation

* Lie flat on your back on your mat or towel, with your knees bent, feet flat on the floor and your arms relaxed at your sides.
* Keeping your hips and bottom on the floor, raise one knee up towards your chest and take hold of the leg lightly behind the knee. Keeping hold of the leg, straighten it towards the ceiling. You may have to lower your leg a little to do this so that the toes are pointing towards the top of the wall rather than the ceiling (fig. below).

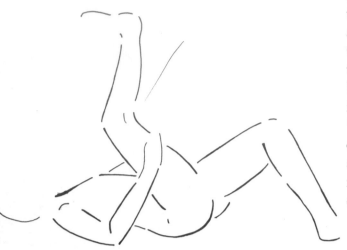

towards the floor, and as you do so, use that energy to draw an imaginary line across the ceiling and slowly down the wall. Once your leg reaches the floor, draw it up to meet the other leg, so that both legs are bent and the soles of the feet are flat on the floor.

* Draw the other leg up towards your chest. Take hold of it lightly and then straighten it towards the ceiling. You are now ready to repeat the exercise with the other leg.

Sequence

* Breathe in and at the same time flex the foot and bend the knee in towards your chest. Continue to hold the working leg lightly (fig. above).
* Breathe out and stretch the heel of the foot up towards the ceiling, straightening the leg as you do so. Send the energy and breath strongly out through the heel of the foot, then point the toes to elongate the foot, and send the energy out through the toes.
* Breathe in and draw the knee to the chest again, flexing the foot.
* Breathe out, straightening the leg up towards the ceiling and push the energy out first through the heel and then the toes.
* Repeat this flexing and stretching sequence four times in total. On the last repetition, keep the raised leg pointing towards the ceiling. Imagine that the energy coming through the leg is travelling way beyond your body and is visible like a laser. Start to slowly lower the straight leg

Notes

* Throughout the exercise check that your chest, upper body and arms are relaxed. If you are able to hold onto the raised leg comfortably without straining and without lifting the upper body off the floor, then try bringing the leg a little higher each time as you straighten it on the 'out' breath.
* Use your arms to exert a gentle, constant pressure on the raised leg, but never pull or jerk the leg with the arms.
* Use the outward flow of the breath to release the muscles, and imagine the leg elongating as the energy travels out through it into the universe.

8 FOOT BOUNCE AND CIRCLE

A strengthening and stretching exercise for the feet, ankles, calves and the backs of the legs.

Preparation

* Sit on the floor on your mat or towel, with your knees bent and feet flat on the floor at a comfortable distance away from the body. Keep your spine long, lift high out of the hips and try to maintain this throughout the exercise. Lightly hug the legs around the thighs or the backs of the knees.

Sequence

* The first part of the exercise focuses on the feet. Using only the strength of the foot, push your right leg off the floor, pushing with the toes and the arch of the foot. Once you have pushed off the floor, lift the leg as high as is comfortable.
* Place the right foot back on the floor and at the same time, push off the floor with the toes and the arch of the left foot, then lift the leg as high as possible.
* Push off the floor and raise the right leg again and at the same time replace the left foot on the floor for balance. Continue pushing off with the feet and lifting alternate legs. Try 20 leg lifts in total.
* Next, raise your right leg and straighten it, supporting the leg with both arms around the thigh or the back of the knee. Hold the leg at a height where you can comfortably straighten it while keeping your spine supported and straight at the base. Imagine the raised leg is very long and extends way beyond your toes. Breathe out and send energy out through the leg. Keep your back alive by consciously directing the breath up and down your spine.
* Still focusing on the energy travelling along the raised leg and beyond, circle the foot ten times in one direction, then reverse and circle ten times in the opposite direction, all the while circling around the line of the energy and breathing normally.
* Slowly lower the right leg and place the foot on the floor. Lift your left leg, supporting it with both arms behind the thigh or around the back of the knee (fig. below).

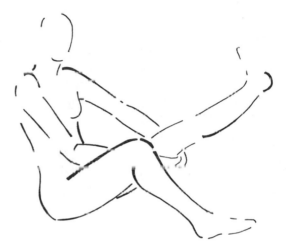

Breathe and with the 'out' breath send energy out through the raised leg and at the same time up through the spine and through the crown of the head. Circle the foot ten times in one direction then ten times in the opposite direction, circling around the outward flowing energy and breathing normally
* Slowly place the left foot back on the floor. Shake out both legs on the floor.

Notes

* The impetus of pushing off the floor with the foot will make the leg lift feel like a bounce or spring. If you cannot feel enough strength in the toes and the arch of the working foot to raise the leg, then use the strength of your leg but focus on the impetus of the movement coming from your feet. Eventually you will begin to feel the isolation of the impetus and to develop sufficient strength in the feet.

9 OUTER THIGH CHAIR PRESS

This is a very effective strengthening and toning exercise for the hips, bottom and outer thighs. Make sure you choose a chair that is relatively sturdy and that can withstand the pressure in this exercise, since the strength of your legs and hips could possibly break a light chair!

Preparation

* Sit on the floor, with the chair facing you. Place your legs between the legs of the chair and sit upright with your legs outstretched. Ideally, the chair legs should make contact with the outside of your shins, just above the ankle bones. Lean back slightly and place your hands on the floor behind you for support. Do not sink down into your shoulders, but keep your spine long. Unlock the elbows (fig. below).

Sequence

* Breathe out and, keeping your legs straight, press outwards with your legs against the chair for a count of ten. Breathe in and out during the count of ten, and imagine you are sending the energy and breath down and out through the legs as you press.
* Release the legs, relax and breathe in. Rest for a moment.
* Breathe out and begin again, pressing against the legs of the chair for a further count of ten. Release.
* Try this ten times in total. The amount of force that you apply is up to you, but do start gently.

Notes

* Once you are familiar with this exercise, try sitting upright, without the support of your hands. If this feels comfortable, reach your arms out at shoulder height towards the chair as you do the exercise. Now focus on the breath travelling out through the five points: through both arms and both feet reaching forwards, and through the top of your head. If you can also manage to visualize a sixth direction, send the breath out down the spine and through the sitting bones into the floor. Reaching forwards with the arms changes the press of the hips and thighs so that you are using different parts of the muscles. Try alternating this position with the supported sitting position.

your feet are touching the chair legs. Lean back a little and place your hands on the floor behind you for support. Keep your spine and neck long and do not sink down into your shoulders. Unlock the elbows.

Sequence

* Press into the chair with the arches of your feet, breathing out over a count of ten and keeping your legs straight. If this breathing is too slow for you, breathe in and out during the count of ten (fig. below).

10 INNER THIGH CHAIR PRESS

A very effective strengthening and toning exercise for the bottom, hips and the inner and upper thighs.

Preparation

* Sit on the floor in front of the chair. Place your feet to either side of the chair and sit upright with legs outstretched. Let your knees fall to the sides so that the soles of

* Breathe in and release the press.
* Press again, breathing out over a count of ten.
* Repeat the exercise about ten times. As with the outer thigh press, the amount of pressure you apply is up to you, but begin gently as it is a deceptively powerful exercise.

Notes

* Focus on the outward flow of energy and breath travelling down the legs, through the feet and out through the toes. Keep the feet soft and not gripped, despite the force. As with the Outer Thigh Chair Press, if you can sit upright comfortably without the support of your hands, reach forwards with the arms at shoulder height. Imagine that the energy travelling through your arms reaches way beyond the chair. Alternate this position from time to time with the supported sitting position.

*11 KNEE LIFTS

This exercise strengthens the legs, hips, stomach and coordinates the breathing.

Preparation

* Stand facing a wall, with your body square to it, feet parallel, and your weight centred over the feet. Release any gripping in your feet and the front of the ankles.
* Place your fingertips or palms lightly on the wall for balance. Take a moment to breathe. Breathe in to start.

Sequence

* With a firm 'out' breath, raise your heels and lift up to half foot, sending the energy and the breath out through the body and down into the earth to form imaginary roots. This position should feel very solid

and balanced.

* On the next 'in' breath, lift your right knee high in front of your body and, at the same time, lower your left heel to the floor, keeping the left leg straight. Don't consciously use any muscle effort to lift the leg, just let the air that is drawn into your body lift the leg up from the kneecap. Be aware of the two different directions of the movement – the downward movement of the supporting left heel and the upward direction of the right knee lift.

* Breathe out, raise onto half foot on the

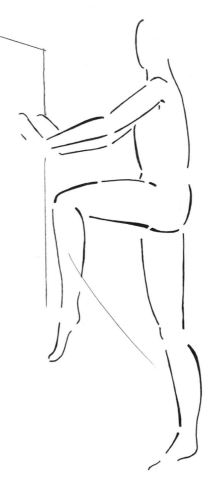

left leg and lower the right leg to meet the left in the half foot position. As the legs meet, send the energy strongly into the earth as before to form stable roots.

* Breathe in and lift the left knee while lowering the right heel to the floor (fig. left). Lift the knee high, using the impulse of the incoming breath.

* Breathe out strongly into the earth as you raise onto half foot on the right leg and bring the left foot to meet it in the half foot position.

* Try 10–12 lifts with alternate knees. Finish on an 'out' breath with the feet together in the half foot position and then slowly lower the heels and breathe naturally.

Notes

* Each time you lower the supporting heel, try to resist the lowering. This will strengthen the feet and legs. Imagine the back of the supporting leg is very long.

* As you lift the knee, keep the body lifted out of the hips. Try not to use any conscious effort to do this, but let the action come from the air that is drawn into the body on the 'in' breath.

*12 FIGURE OF EIGHT

This exercise develops mobility and strength in the hips and torso. The figure of eight is the movement performed by the knee of the working leg.

Preparation

* Stand with your left side to the wall and reach your left arm out just below shoulder height. Place your palm firmly on the wall for support and place your right arm out to the side for balance.

* Raise your right knee up in front of you and then open it out to your right side, letting the lower part of the leg hang down naturally from the knee. Check that your weight is spread evenly through your left supporting foot and that your left leg is very slightly bent, not locked.

Sequence

* Breathe out and turn the right knee inwards towards the supporting leg so that the foot and calf point out to the right side. Lead with the knee and pass the right leg in front of the left leg, turning the hips and torso towards the left to allow this movement to happen.

* Breathe in and lift the right knee up in front of you (fig. overleaf left). Turn it and open it out so that the calf and foot are pointing directly down, then lift the knee high up to the right side.

* Breathe out and take the right knee directly down so that the right foot and calf pass down behind the left leg and cross over to the left side of it .

* Breathe in and lift the knee up directly behind you (fig. overleaf right), then bring it forwards and high up to the side. You have just completed one figure of eight with the leg.

* Try six to eight in total on this side. On the last repetition, after the knee comes

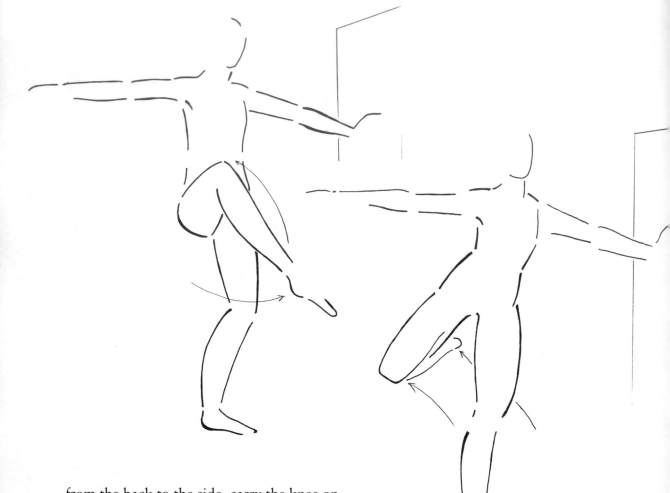

from the back to the side, carry the knee on in front of you, then lower the leg to the floor.

* Turn around and extend your right arm out just below shoulder height. Place your right palm flat against the wall. Lift your left knee up to the front, then open it out to the side and let the lower leg hang down naturally. Check that your weight is distributed evenly over your right foot and then repeat the exercise with the left knee.

Notes

* Keep the working leg relaxed in the hip joint throughout the exercise. Imagine you are lifting and leading only with the knee, and visualize the figure of eight that you are drawing.

Figure of Eight Variation

When you are very comfortable with the original exercise, try integrating the upper body into the exercise by coordinating it with the movement of the knee. The basic exercise remains the same.

* Start as before. This time as you breathe out and carry the knee across in front of you, turning the hips as before, slowly bend the supporting leg, while curving your right arm across in front of the body and curving your spine over the raised knee.
* As you breathe in and carry the knee forwards and then out to the side, open out the arm and the body to mirror the movement of the knee and, at the same time, straighten the supporting leg.
* As you breathe out and take the leg down behind the supporting leg, follow that movement with the arm, making the same kind of fluid figure of eight movement behind the body with the arm. Keep your spine upright and keep the supporting leg straight.

Notes

* Adding the upper body and the arm movement to the exercise should give it the feeling of opening and closing. The bend on the supporting leg happens only on the forward part of the figure of eight.

*13 TRAVELLING KNEE LIFTS

This exercise develops your sense of balance and coordination as well as strengthening the hips, stomach and back.

Preparation

* Stand in the centre of your exercise space, with your feet together. Breathe for a moment, using the image of the Energy Fountain (see page 13).
* Find a point at eye level to focus on during the exercise. Lift your arms wide to the side, just below shoulder height. Hold the arms just in front of the body line so that you are aware of them out of the corner of each eye. Turn your feet out to about 45 degrees, keeping your heels touching. Relax your feet. Check that the whole of each foot is in contact with the floor and that your weight is distributed evenly over them.
* Send the 'out' breath down your arms and out to the sides of your space. Imagine you are reaching out to a distant wall on each side, and feel the two-way pull through the arms opening your chest.

Travelling forwards

* Lift your right knee up to the side, sliding your right foot up the side of the supporting leg to touch the knee. Then bounce the right knee higher up towards your body, sending the right foot out away from the knee. Let the foot hang down naturally from the ankle (fig. overleaf).
* Place your right foot on the floor in front

91

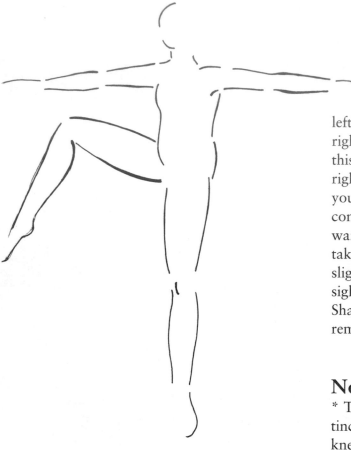

Travelling backwards

* After completing your travelling knee lifts forwards, the last foot to be placed down will be the left. Begin travelling backwards by picking up the left knee, sliding the left foot up the supporting leg to touch the right knee. Bounce the left knee higher and this time place the foot down behind the right foot, transferring your weight onto your left foot. Pick up the right knee and continue the travelling knee lifts backwards, alternating left and right knees and taking care to keep the arms fluid and slightly in front of the body, just within eyesight. Do six knee lifts and then finish. Shake out the arms and upper body to remove any stiffness or holding.

Notes

* The rhythm of the exercise has three distinct points: lift to touch the side of the knee, bounce higher, place the foot on the floor. Try to coordinate the breath with the movement. Choose the rhythm of the breath that feels most natural to you and that helps the exercise feel effortless. For example: breathe in as you lift and then bounce the knee, and breathe out as you place the foot on the floor.
* Throughout this exercise keep lifting the upper body high out of the hips and legs. Imagine the upper body is gliding effortlessly and independently as you step.

of the left. Transfer the weight of the body evenly onto your right foot so that you have taken a step forwards.

* Lift your left knee up high to the side, sliding the left foot up the side of the right leg to touch the knee. Bounce the left knee higher, sending the left foot out to the side so that the leg is bent at a right angle.

* Place your left foot in front of the right and transfer your weight onto your left foot.

* Continue with alternate knee lifts so that you travel forwards. Do six in total then move on to the next part of the exercise.

Travelling Knee Lifts Variation

Do the original exercise first and then add the following variation.

* Stand with your upper body held high. Turn your toes out and then put your right foot slightly behind the left foot to start.
* In a smooth movement, lift the right knee up from behind, take it up and out to the side, then place it down in front of the right foot. The whole movement is an arc. The lower part of the leg should be relaxed so that the leg is bent naturally at an approximate right angle.
* Smoothly transfer the weight to the right foot, then lift the left knee to draw an arc up and over to the side. Place the left foot down in front, smoothly transfer the weight and continue lifting alternate knees.
* Do six travelling forwards, then reverse by lifting your left foot first and do six travelling backwards. The backward arc from front to back is a little more difficult to perform, so focus clearly on a fixed point at eye level. Breathe in the direction of the Energy Fountain, lifting the weight out of the hips and carrying the body lightly. Carry the arms slightly in front of the body and be aware of them out of the corner of your eyes. Try to coordinate your breathing with the movement as described in the original exercise.
* To finish, shake out the arms and upper body and relax.

*14 HIP FLEXOR

A powerful stretch for the stomach, hips and whole of the legs.

Preparation

* Stand in the centre of your exercise space, with your feet as wide apart as your hips. Breathe and release any tension in the upper body.
* Breathe out and crouch down so that your heels come off the floor. Curve your spine over your legs and place the palms of your hands in front of you on the floor.

Sequence

* Breathe in and place your right leg straight out behind you on the floor with the heel raised. Lower the heel of your left leg and place your hands to either side of the left leg for support (fig. below).

* Breathe out and very gently press into your right heel for a count of ten, feeling the stretch in the front of the right thigh and hip and in the right calf.
* Breathe in and slowly straighten your left leg so that your body is now between your straight legs. Lower the right heel towards the floor – it will not reach the floor completely (fig. below).

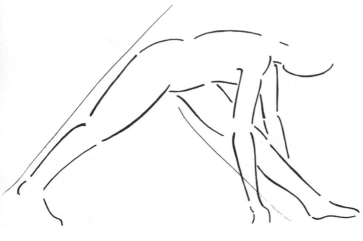

* Breathe out and gently press the body forwards over your straight left leg, curving your spine over towards the knee for a count of ten. Use the image of the outward-flowing breath to dissipate the stiffness in the back of the leg. Use the tips of your fingers on the floor to either side of you for support.
* Breathe in and flex the left foot up towards you so that your weight is resting on your left heel.
* Breathe out and gently press over the leg for another count of ten. Feel the increased stretch up the back of the left leg, and use the 'out' breath to clear the stiffness.
* Breathe in and place your left toes on the floor and slowly bend your left leg so that your body shifts forwards again. This time bend your right leg and put the knee on the floor, bringing your spine more upright.
* Breathe out and gently press forwards for a count of ten, opening the right hip.
* Breathe in and curve over your left knee. Place your hands on the floor for support and bring the right leg in to join the left so that you are once again crouching with heels off the floor.
* Breathe out, relax the legs and release the shoulders before starting again.
* Breathe in and send your left leg out directly behind you. Curve forwards over your bent right leg and place your hands on the floor to either side of the leg for support. Then continue as before.

Notes

* Note that in this exercise any change of position is accompanied by the 'in' breath so that the body is lifted by the breath and the limb is carried carefully into its new position. Each pressing and stretching moment uses the release of the 'out' breath to extend the movement and dissipate tension and toxins. Never move rapidly into or out of the stretches but always control these movements.

*15 SITTING SIDE STRETCH

A strengthening and stretching exercise for the legs, hips and waist.

Preparation

* Sit on the floor with your legs bent in front of you and the soles of your feet on the floor. Straighten and open your legs at approximately a 90-degree angle so that the legs point to the corners of the room. If you cannot sit with the spine upright, bring your legs a little closer together.

* Warm up the hip joints for a moment by making four small circles with the torso in one direction and then four in the opposite direction. Imagine that your legs are very long and send energy through them out to the corners of the room. Try to maintain this image throughout the exercise.

* Breathe in and elongate the neck and spine to begin.

Sequence

* Breathe out for eight counts, curving your head and upper body forwards between your legs. Let your arms and shoulders hang relaxed between your legs. Release the spine over a little more with each count of the 'out' breath.

* Breathe in and use the breath to inflate the spine vertebra by vertebra and uncurl to upright.

* Breathe out and relax.

* Breathe in and raise the right arm in an arc, reaching out wide to the side and then upwards until the arm points directly towards the ceiling and is next to your ear. Lengthen the spine and neck. Place the back of your left hand relaxed on the floor between your legs or by your side for support.

* Breathe out over eight counts and reach up and over your head towards the top of the left wall, leaning your body directly over the left leg (fig. below). Reach a little further over the left leg with each count as

you release into the stretch, sending the energy way out beyond the body through the raised arm and through both legs.

* Breathe in and, keeping the right arm high by your ear, turn your upper body to face your left leg.

* Breathe out over eight counts and reach

forwards with both arms, over the left leg (fig. below). Send energy out through the arms, beyond the toes of the left leg,

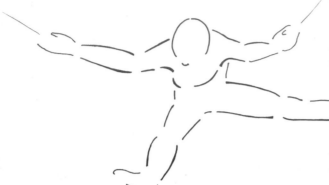

releasing more into the stretch with each count.

* Breathe in, relax and curve your spine down over your left leg. Bring your curved body to the centre between your legs and then use the breath to inflate the spine and uncurl to upright.

* Begin again. Breathe out over eight counts and curve forwards. Try to release the upper body between your legs.

* Breathe in to uncurl to upright, then breathe out and relax.

* Breathe in and raise your left arm in an arc wide to the side, then upwards by your ear.

* Breathe out over eight counts, reaching up and over the right leg, placing the back of the right hand on the floor between your legs or by your side for support. Continue with the stretches as before.

* To finish, breathe in and curve your spine over your right leg. Bring your body to the front to hang between your legs then uncurl

the spine as before. Shake out your legs on the floor, gradually moving them together in front of you. Rub the backs of the legs vigorously before going on to your next exercise.

Notes

* Throughout the exercise, keep the idea of the legs being long, elongating out of the hips and reaching out far beyond the body. As you reach over the left leg, send energy out through the right leg and vice versa. This helps to balance you and also strengthens the hips.

*16 SITTING FLEX

An effective stretching and strengthening exercise for the legs, hips and stomach.

Preparation

* Sit on the floor with your knees bent in front of you and soles of the feet flat on the floor.

* Move your feet apart to 45 degrees and then stretch your legs out. Keeping your back upright from the base of the spine, adjust your legs by taking them as wide apart as is comfortable.

* To warm up the hips before you begin, gently circle the upper body. Make four small circles in one direction and then four in the opposite direction. You will feel this

stretching and working the hip joints and the muscles in the back of the legs.

* Return to the upright position in the centre and begin.

Sequence

* Breathe in and, leaving the heel of your right foot where it is, bend the right knee and flex the toes up towards you. At the same time, use the breath to draw your right arm up above your head as if describing the upward path of the energy.
* Breathe out firmly and straighten your right leg and elongate the foot, sending the breath out a long way from the body, through the right leg and toes. At the same time reach out over your right leg and direct the breath out through the arm and fingers towards the corner of the room.
* With the 'in' breath, draw your body back up to centre. Relax the right arm and draw the left arm up to above your head as if describing the energy entering the body. At the same time, flex your left foot up towards you and bend the knee, leaving the heel where it is (fig. right).

* With the 'out' breath send the energy and breath out strongly through the left leg and foot, straightening the leg and elongating the foot. At the same time reach out over the leg, sending energy out to the corner with the left arm.
* Continue as before, alternating right and left. Try 12 in total.
* To come out of this exercise, finish on an 'in' breath, drawing the body back up to centre, but leave the arms relaxed and down. Shake the legs out on the floor and bring them slowly together in front of you as you shake them. Rub vigorously any muscles that you can feel have been stretched, particularly the back of the thighs.

Notes

* Try to establish an energetic, coordinated rhythm to the breathing and movement that feels good to do. Use the working arm to give a shape to the movements. It gathers up the energy and then sends it out to the corners of your space. Each time you breathe out, imagine your legs are growing and elongating as you straighten them and reach out and over with the arm.

Sitting Flex Variation

This is a more powerful version which creates a greater flow of energy and a greater stretch, so make sure you are sufficiently warmed up before starting.

* Do the original exercise as before about eight times, alternating left and right, and then put the left and right movements together so that you do them simultaneously as follows.
* Breathe in and draw both arms up above your head. Keep your spine and neck long and your shoulders relaxed. At the same time, flex both feet up towards you and bend both knees.

* Breathe out and feel like a wonderful open star sending energy out in every direction as you open your arms wide and straighten your legs, elongating the feet and shooting energy to the corners of your space through both legs and both arms. Also, if you can, imagine sending energy firmly through the spine, through the head and down into the floor to connect you. Feel the energy through the spine keeping you very strong in the centre of your body and preventing you from being pulled off-balance to either side. This position should feel energized yet centred and balanced, with a complete elongation and opening of the body.
* Try four to six repetitions.

Notes

* The coordination of the movement, breath and energy images may appear a little complex at first. Be patient and start by familiarizing yourself with the mechanical coordination. Once you are familiar with the mechanics of the exercise, you can begin to add the energy images and directions until you are able to hold all the ideas in your Mind's Eye at once.

STEP 4

STRENGTHENING

1 CYCLING

This exercise strengthens the stomach and legs.

Preparation
* Lie down on the floor on your mat or towel, with your arms relaxed by your sides. Lift both knees up towards your chest and raise your head off the floor. Focus on a point in front of you, several feet away across the room, about six inches (15 cm) off the floor.

Sequence
* Extend one leg straight out so that it is just off the floor. Aim to reach the point of

focus with the energy you send out through the leg and foot (fig. below).
* Draw the leg back to your chest and extend the other leg out straight, just off the

floor, aiming to send energy to your focus point.
* Continue alternating legs and aim to do

20 leg extensions in total. Control the extension of the legs so that you do not jar the knees as the leg straightens.

* To finish, bring both knees into the chest and hug them close to the body. Release your stomach muscles as you breathe in this position.

Notes

* Try to keep the breath relaxed and regular and coordinate it with the movement. For example, breathe out over two leg extensions right and left, then breathe in over two extensions.
* Keep your head raised the whole time and your eyes focused on the point in front of you. Your arms and upper body stay relaxed throughout.

Cycling Variation

* Try ten leg extensions as above, sending the energy out through the toes to the point of focus, then do ten more, this time flexing the foot as you extend the leg. Feel the energy travelling down the back of the leg and strongly out through the heel to the point of focus

2 SPIRAL SLIDE

A rhythmic strengthening exercise for the stomach and the back.

Preparation

* Sit on the floor on your mat or towel, with your knees bent and feet flat on the floor at a comfortable distance away from the body. The legs should stay in this position throughout the exercise to act as an anchor point. Try to consciously relax them and let the upper body do all the work.
* Breathe and elongate the spine, lifting up out of the hips. Relax the shoulders and arms and leave them by your sides.

Sequence

* Breathe out and curve your head to your chest. Slowly roll down your spine towards the floor, vertebra by vertebra, beginning with your lower back and finishing as your head uncurls and rests on the floor. At the same time, bend your arms and curl them by your sides, up past your ears and then extend them overhead just off the floor.
* No sooner than your head has touched the floor, use the 'in' breath to curl up to the upright position. Begin by curving your head forwards to your chest and then continue to curl your spine towards your knees. At the same time, bend your arms and bring them to your ears and then extend them out in front of you as you sit up.
* Breathe out and relax.
* Now breathe in and do a 'backstroke' swimming movement with the right arm by raising the arm up in front of you, passing it overhead and then placing the tips of the fingers on the floor a little way behind you.
* Breathe out and, keeping the arm straight, slide it directly away behind you

on the floor placing some weight first on the fingertips and then on the palm. As you do this, your body will automatically turn to face the right side (fig. below). Let your

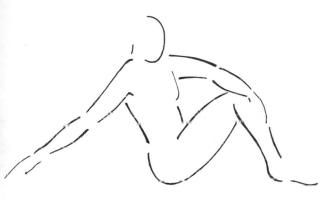

body follow the arm and, as your arm reaches directly overhead, allow your body to open out and lie flat on the floor. In a smooth movement, swap the arms over by bringing your right arm from overhead to by your side and at the same time lift the left arm from your side to over your head. The two arms should pass each other.

* Breathe in and use the breath to draw your body up, lifting the ribcage and the middle of the back off the floor first. As you lift up, your body will turn to face the left. Support the movement by sliding on the palm and then on the fingertips of the left hand with your arm outstretched behind you (fig. below). As you come up to the upright position, bring your body to face front and leave the left arm by your side.

* In a continuous movement reverse the slide. Breathe in and make a 'backstroke' movement with the left arm, lifting it up in front, then carrying it overhead and down behind your body.

* Breathe out and allow your body to turn and face the left as you slide down on the fingertips of the left hand, keeping the arm straight. When the arm is directly overhead, roll flat onto your back and swap arms by lifting your right arm over your head and taking your left arm down to your side.

* Breathe in and raise your body up from the middle of the back, turning to face the right side and sliding on the palm of the right hand as you rise. As you come to sit upright, bring your body to face front and let your right arm relax by your side.

* Sit up very tall and carry both arms up in front of you to form a circle at chest height.

* Breathe out and open the chest and shoulders to the ceiling. Gently tilt your head back as a natural extension of the spine.

* Breathe in and draw the spine upright.

* Breathe out and relax, the arms ready to begin again.

* Try the whole exercise four times in total.

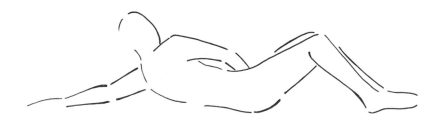

Notes

* If you find the first roll up or down difficult to do smoothly, reach forwards with your arms at shoulder height and focus on sending a continuous flow of energy out through the raised arms as you roll up and down. This will help you to overcome any weak points in the roll.

* It may take a little while to familiarize yourself with the coordination of the movements in this exercise, in particular the part where you raise the body on a spiral, so be patient. When you are familiar with the movements it is a very beautiful exercise to do. Focus on the fluidity and continuity of the movements and try to develop a confident rhythm. Concentrate on the flow and rhythm of the arm and slide movements rather than on the muscular effort involved in raising and lowering your spine. The muscular strength will develop naturally.

3 CURL UP

An exercise to strengthen the stomach.

Preparation

* Lie on the floor on your mat or towel, with your arms relaxed by your sides and your knees bent, feet flat on the floor. Breathe. Feel the spine very long and straight, and release the neck and jaw.

Sequence

* On an 'out' breath, curl your head and shoulders up off the floor, curling smoothly up the spine and lifting high enough so that the upper back is just off the floor. As you lift up, reach straight out towards the far wall in front of you with both arms, raising the arms on the outside of the knees. Hold and breathe out for a count of ten. Focus on sending the energy and breath out through the arms to the far wall in front of you (fig. below).

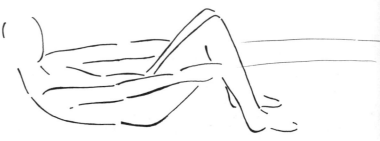

* Breathe in and slowly uncurl the spine back down until you are lying flat.
* Breathe out and release the stomach and the neck muscles.
* Breathe in and elongate the spine, then begin again.
* This is quite a strenuous movement, so start with just three repetitions and gradually work your way up to five.

Notes

* As you become stronger, aim to lift a little higher. But always keep the small of the back in contact with the floor. Use the reach with the arms and the image of the energy flowing out through them to raise you. Focus on the idea of energy flowing

through the entire body and beyond, and aim to keep the front of the body fluid by using the movement of the 'out' breath during the lifting.

Curl Up Variation

This variation is much more strenuous than the original exercise so only attempt this if the original exercise has become easy and you can do it without any tension in the upper body, chest and neck. Later, you could try alternating it with the original.

* Lie on the floor as before with knees bent. Breathe for a moment, elongating the spine and neck.

* Raise both knees together towards your chest. Release the legs in the hip joints and just let the legs remain above your body supported by their natural weight, without any conscious effort on your part.

* Now do the exercise as before, curling your head and shoulders off the floor and reaching your arms straight out in front, but leave your bent legs where they are. Your back will not lift as high off the floor as in the original exercise. Breathe out over ten counts. Keep the breathing soft and fluid and allow it to flow continuously through the body and beyond, carrying toxins and waste with it and clearing the muscles.

* Breathe in and slowly uncurl the spine down to the floor.

* As with the original exercise work your way gradually up to five repetitions.

4 SHOULDER STANDS

This series of shoulder stand exercises are performed with the body supported on the shoulders in order to use gravity as a strengthening aid.

Preparation for all shoulder stand exercises:
* Lie flat on your back on the floor on your mat or towel, with your arms at your sides, knees bent and soles of the feet flat on the floor.
* Breathe for a moment and feel the whole of your back in contact with the floor. As you breathe in, elongate the spine and the neck.
* Now, bring both knees up to your chest. Carry the legs on over your head, gently rolling your spine off the floor until your knees are above your head, with toes pointing towards the floor beyond your head. Bend your elbows and place your hands on the middle of your back for support. Slowly raise your bent legs vertically above you. Adjust your hands if necessary for maximum support. When you feel balanced, slowly straighten the legs so that they point towards the ceiling. Breathe.

SHOULDER STAND 1: CYCLING

Exercise to increase hip flexibility and to strengthen the legs and stomach.

* Begin up on your shoulders with your legs together and vertical and your feet parallel.
* Draw one knee down towards the chest and send energy strongly through the straight leg upwards, way beyond you (fig. left).

* Now begin cycling. Unfold the bent leg forwards over your head and then circle it up into the air, sending energy out through it. At the same time, let the straight leg bend and drop down behind the body, then draw it through towards your chest. Alternate the drawing through of the legs to the chest with the unfolding action so that the legs move in a cycling motion. Take care to control all the movements. Carry the legs, and do not simply let them drop with gravity.
* Try 20 in total. Come out of this exercise as described below.

Coming out of the shoulder stands
* To come out of all of the shoulder stand exercises, breathe in and slowly bend your knees towards your head, keeping the legs together. Let the toes drop over towards the floor beyond your head.
* Using your hands for support, slowly roll your spine down until the whole of your back is in contact with the floor and your knees are bent above your chest. Then slowly lower both legs together until the feet are flat on the floor.
* If you want to get up off the floor, roll over to your right side with your back curved around your knees. Then, using your arms to assist, come up onto your knees and then up to standing.

SHOULDER STAND 2: TWIST

Exercise to tone the waist and the outer thighs.

* Begin up on your shoulders, with your legs touching and pointing directly upwards. Take a moment to breathe. With a firm 'out' breath, send energy up and out through the legs into the universe.
* Breathe in and draw your knees down towards your head. Control the lowering of the knees over four counts. Keeping your knees together and your head straight, spiral in the waist and touch your right cheek

SHOULDER STAND 3: SCISSORS

Exercise to strengthen and stretch the inner thigh muscles.

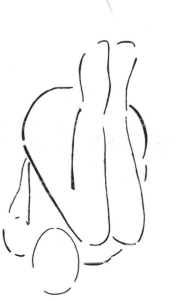

* Begin up on your shoulders as before, with your legs together and pointing directly up into the air. Turn your toes out to about 45 degrees so that your knees are facing the corners of the room.
* Send energy firmly up through both legs, elongating the feet. In small, rapid movements, criss-cross the feet by crossing the right foot in front of the left and then the left foot in front of the right. Continue alternating right and left in small scissorlike movements, sending energy upwards the whole time. Do about 20 in total (fig below).

with the outside of the left knee (fig. above).
* Breathe out and control the movement as you straighten your legs vertically. Send the breath and energy firmly upwards, elongating the legs. Relax your neck and shoulders.
* Breathe in and draw the legs down towards your head over four counts, then spiral in the waist so that the outside of the right knee touches your left cheek.
* Breathe out and straighten your legs vertically as before, sending the energy out through the feet and elongating the legs. The legs should remain touching from the ankle to the thigh throughout the exercise.
* Try ten sets of bending and straightening in total, spiralling to alternate sides. Come out of this exercise as described earlier (see page 104) for all the shoulder stand exercises.

* Next, keeping the legs straight, breathe in and slowly separate the legs, opening them as far as is comfortable so that the feet point towards the corners of the room.

* Breathe out and relax the leg muscles, allowing gravity to stretch the legs a little. Do not bounce or force the legs further apart.

* Breathe in and bend the knees so that the soles of the feet meet each other and then slowly straighten the legs to the vertical position with the feet and heels touching.

* Begin again with the scissor-like movements of criss-crossing the legs. Try the whole sequence three or four times in total.

* Come out of this exercise as described earlier (see page 104) for all the shoulder stand exercises.

to each side as they bend. This should exert a constant pressure on the tops of the feet (fig. below).

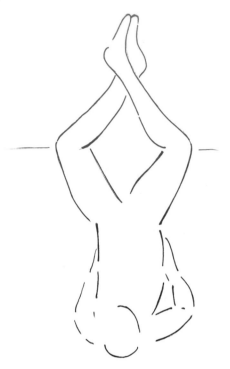

SHOULDER STAND 4: ISOMETRIC PULL

Exercise to strengthen the inner and outer thighs and the ankles.

* Begin up on your shoulders with your legs together and pointing directly upwards. Turn your toes out to about 45 degrees then cross them at the ankles. Bend your knees a little so that the knees face the corners of the room, and press the tops of the feet together.

* With a sustained 'out' breath, very slowly bend your knees, drawing them down towards you. At the same time imagine that your knees are being pulled away

* When your legs are bent as far as is comfortable, breathe in and release the imaginary pull to the sides momentarily, but keep the ankles crossed.

* Breathe out and resume the imaginary pull to the sides so that you feel pressure against the tops of the feet and, at the same time, slowly straighten your legs. Keep hold of the pulling image so that you maintain a constant, gentle pressure throughout the straightening.

* When the legs are straight, breathe in and release the pulling image, cross the ankles over the other way, then on an 'out' breath begin again by slowly bending the legs with a constant pull to the sides.

* Try four complete sets of bending and straightening, alternating the foot that is crossed in front. The image of pulling the knees to the sides while they are actually held in place by the feet works the inner and outer thigh muscles and the ankles.
* Come out of this exercise as described earlier (see page 104) for all the shoulder stand exercises.

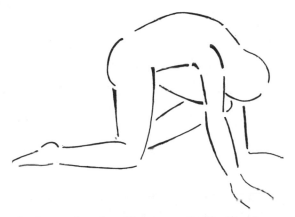

5 ALL FOURS LEG LIFTS

A whole body strengthening exercise.

Preparation

* Get down on the floor on your mat or towel and position yourself on your hands and knees. Place your hands directly under your shoulders and your knees directly under your hips. Imagine your spine is very long and horizontal with energy travelling along it in both directions and continuing horizontally way beyond the body. Breathe in and lift one knee off the floor to begin.

Sequence

* Breathe out and curve your head in towards your body while bringing your knee up towards your nose. Curve your spine up to the ceiling as much as possible (fig. top right).
* Breathe in and elongate your body, then arch it by opening your chest and head up towards the ceiling. At the same time swing

the knee down and out to the back of you then up, as if the toes were being pulled directly up into the air (fig. below).

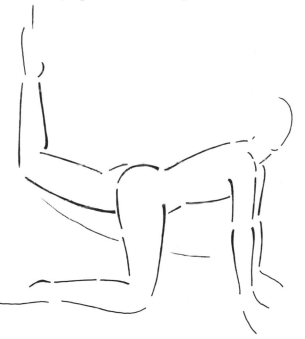

* Breathe out and curve your spine again, drawing the knee to meet the nose and repeat.
* Repeat ten times, then place the knee back on the floor and breathe, sending the breath the length of the spine.
* Repeat with the other leg.

Notes

* The breathing pattern described above is the most natural one for this sequence, but if you reverse the pattern, you may find that it helps you to lift the leg higher. To do this, breathe in and draw the knee and head towards each other, expanding and curving your spine and chest with the incoming air. Then breathe out firmly through the top of the head and out through the raised leg, sending the air out through the leg and out into the universe. Use whichever breathing pattern feels most helpful to you.

All Fours Curve and Stretch, Step 5 (page 119) would be a good exercise to move on to after this one.

6 LEG CIRCLES

This exercise strengthens and tones the backs of the legs and the bottom.

Preparation

* Lie face down on the floor on your mat or towel. Fold your arms in front of your head, palms flat on the floor, and place your forehead or chin on your hands.
* Breathe for a moment, elongating your spine and neck. Relax your upper body and shoulders and elongate your feet. As you breathe, send energy out through the legs, imagining them to be as long as possible.

Sequence

* Maintaining the image of very long legs, breathe in and lift your right leg just off the floor, no higher than six inches (15 cm), reaching a long way from the body with the raised leg.
* Now do ten small outward circles with the right leg. Imagine your toes are drawing the circles on a distant wall. Breathe out for five circles and breathe in for five circles (fig. below).

* Breathe out and lower the leg to the floor, lengthening the leg as you lower it.

* Again imagining the leg is very long, breathe in and lift the left leg just off the floor. Reach out with the toes to a far wall behind you and make ten small outward circles with the leg, breathing out for five circles then breathing in for five circles.

* Breathe out and lengthen the left leg further as you slowly lower it to the floor.

* Repeat, lifting the right leg first and then the left, but this time reverse the direction of the circle so that you circle inwards.

* Try four complete sets in total.

* To come out of this exercise, use your hands to push back onto your knees, then curve your spine and sit back on your heels, curving your upper body over your knees, your arms extended out in front to stretch the spine. Stay here for a moment and breathe out. Then with an 'in' breath, uncurl the spine to upright and come up to standing.

Notes

* It really does not matter in which direction you start the circles so long as you alternate the directions of the circles.

*7 SWINGING YOUR WEIGHT

A very energized exercise for the whole body which uses the impetus of the breath and the natural weight of the body.

Preparation

* Sit on the floor on your mat or towel with your spine upright, knees bent and feet flat on the floor.

Sequence

* Breathe out firmly and swing your arms and upper body forwards over your legs. As you do so, allow the legs to drop and straighten with the weight of the body, and swing your arms out directly in front. As you swing down, send the energy way out beyond the body through the arms and legs (fig. below).

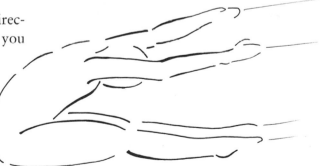

* With the 'in' breath, inflate and lift the upper body and, leaving your legs where they are, swing the upper body upright, carrying your arms straight above your head

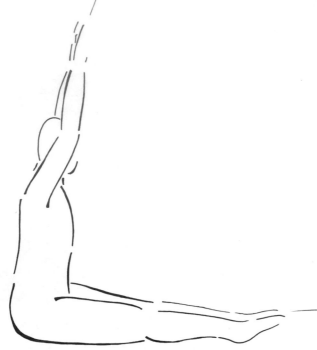

(fig. above).

* Breathe out and let your body and out-stretched arms fall straight forwards again towards your legs. Keep the arms and spine very long.

* Breathe in and draw the knees up towards the chest, as if gathering up energy into your body (fig. below). Sit upright

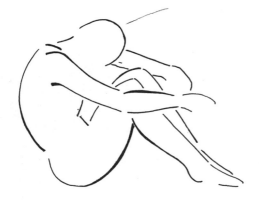

again in the starting position ready to begin again.

* Repeat this four-breath swinging cycle three times.

* Now, leave your legs where they are, breathe out and roll down your spine towards the floor, vertebra by vertebra, keeping the spine very long. You should hardly reach the floor, when the 'in' breath picks you up again, curling your spine up, with head leading. Reach forwards with both arms as you rise until you are sitting upright in the starting position ready to begin again with the four-breath cycle.

* Repeat the three, four-breath swinging cycle, followed by a two-breath roll down and up. Try the whole exercise three times in total.

Notes

* Try to find your own rhythm for the swinging movements of the body. Join all the movements fluidly together, following the rise and fall of the breath. When you become familiar with the movement pattern, try to have a sense of the breath lifting and releasing you so that your body is simply following its impetus. Imagine your body is dancing around like clothes on a clothes line, lifting and falling as they are animated with gusts of air.

* If you find it difficult to roll up the spine, use your hands on the floor to help you up, but try to maintain the fluidity of the movement.

*8 TWISTER

This is a very effective strengthening exercise for the stomach, waist and back.

Preparation

* Lie on your back on the floor on your mat or towel and place your arms out wide on the floor so that they are level with your shoulders. Spread and release your shoulder blades and take a moment to breathe through your spine, legs and outstretched arms.
* Lift your knees up until they are above your hips to begin. Keeping your upper body still and relaxed, breathe in and prepare to swing your bent legs and hips.

Sequence

* With the 'out' breath, twist in the waist and swing the left knee over to face the right wall, without letting the leg touch the floor. Let your right leg swing down so that it is underneath the left leg, and the right thigh is pointing straight down from the hips. Keep both legs off the floor at all times (fig. below).

* Breathe in and swing the left leg back up to the centre above your hips. Bring the right knee up to join it so that the hips and spine are momentarily straight.
* Breathe out and swing the left leg over and down to the left, until the left thigh is pointing straight down from the hip. Let the right leg follow over to the left (fig. above), until the knee is pointing directly to the side.
* Breathe in and twist to the right in the waist and bring the hips straight so that both knees are centred above the body.
* Continue rhythmically swinging from side to side, keeping the legs off the floor. Try ten initially and gradually work up to 20 over the next few months.
* To finish, bring both knees to the chest and hug them close, stretching out the lower spine and releasing the stomach.

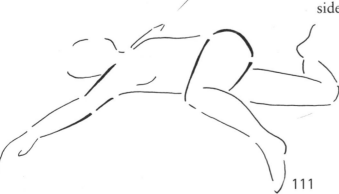

Notes

* During the exercise focus on relaxing the upper body and sending energy out through it across the floor. Relax your chest and the front of the neck, and release any gripping in the hands. Send the breath out along the floor, through the arms and through the top of the head. Imagine each end of your spine continues along the length of the floor, through your sitting bones and through your head. The legs and hips simply rotate and twist around the spine which remains constant.

*9 PELVIC PUSH UP

This exercise develops strength and mobility in the hips, lower back, spine and legs.

Preparation

* Sit on the floor on your mat or towel, with your knees bent in front of you and soles of the feet flat on the floor. Breathe out and, lifting your upper body out of the hips, curve your head to your chest and roll down your spine until you are lying on the floor.
* Breathe for a moment and feel the whole spine in contact with the floor, arms relaxed by your sides. Throughout this exercise keep your shoulders, chest and neck consciously relaxed and let the lower body do all the work.
* Breathe in to begin and lift your forearms up to form a right angle, elbows on the floor.

Sequence

* Breathe out and curl your pelvis up towards the ceiling. You will feel your lower back press into the floor at this point. Press into the feet and lift your hips off the floor completely. Gently press the hips upwards towards the ceiling as high as is comfortable, arching your back. During the upward press of the hips, bring your hands down and slowly press down to the floor with the palms of both hands, as if pressing the breath out with that movement (fig. below).

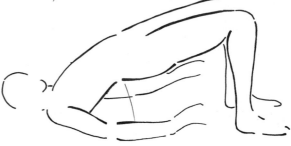

* Breathe in and curl the pelvis up towards the ceiling again, curving your spine, then slowly lower your spine, starting at the top of the ribcage, curling it down vertebra by vertebra until the whole back is in contact with the floor. As you lower the spine, mirror the movement of the 'in' breath by drawing your hands slowly up to right angles again, as if drawing the breath in with this movement. Lastly, straighten your pelvis so that you are lying flat on the floor.
* Continue raising and lowering the spine, using the breath. Try ten in total. On the last one, hold the upward press on the 'out'

breath for a count of ten, then breathe in, curl the pelvis and slowly roll your spine down to the floor.

Notes

* This exercise should be performed very slowly, keeping all the movements controlled. Press a little higher with each 'out' breath, but do not push up further than is comfortable for your spine. The forearms perform a continuous contrary motion to the hips and pelvis that mirrors the movement of the breath.

*10 PELVIC LIFT

A strengthening exercise for the stomach which also massages the hips and lower spine. Make sure you use a towel or mat for this exercise as it can be a little hard on the vertebrae if you are bony.

Preparation

* Lie down on the floor or your mat or towel, with your knees bent and soles of the feet flat on the floor.
* Breathe in and out the length of the spine and release the back muscles. Feel the whole back in contact with the floor.
* Place your arms by your sides, palms on the floor. Breathe in and lift both knees up towards your chest. Relax the hip joints, and begin.

Sequence

* Breathe out and, keeping your knees bent and relaxed above your chest, lift them up towards your nose, curling your pelvis and lower spine off the floor (fig. below).

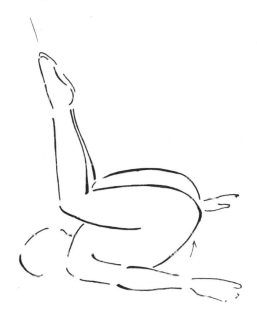

* Breathe in and control the lowering of the spine back to the floor, keeping your knees relaxed above your body.
* Try this slow lifting and lowering movement about ten times. You will find that the chest, neck and arms want to do the work of the stomach muscles, so throughout the exercise check that your chest and the front of your neck are without tension.
* Finish with the knees relaxed above the body, and relax the hip joints and stomach. Feel your whole back in contact with the floor, then go on to the second half of the exercise.
* Breathing naturally, trace a circle with your knees. Begin with the knees above your chest. Carry them slowly to one side,

then down and away from the body, keeping the feet off the floor, then up to the other side and back above the chest. Keep the knees touching at all times.

* Take four circles in one direction, then reverse and do four circles in the opposite direction. The larger the circles, the greater the work for the stomach muscles, so begin with quite small circles. Feel the floor massaging the small of the back and the hips as you circle. Keep your chest, arms and neck released throughout.

* To finish, hug the knees to the chest for a moment, breathe out and release the stomach and spine. To get up, roll onto your right side and then come up to standing.

*11 'ON THE WALK' LEG LIFTS

A strengthening exercise for the hips, bottom and the backs of the thighs. The 'on the walk' position also stretches the hips.

Preparation

* Sit on the floor on your mat or towel, with your knees bent in front of you and soles of the feet flat on the floor. Place your hands to either side of you on the floor for support.

* To get into the 'on the walk' position, drop both knees onto the floor to the left side. Now separate the knees. Take the right knee directly out to the right side and bring the left knee forwards so that it points directly out in front of you. Move the feet out a little so that the legs almost form right angles. Release your hips and keep your spine long. Relax your shoulders, and begin.

Sequence

* Shift the weight of the body slightly to the left, supporting yourself with your left hand on the floor.

* Breathe in and lift your right leg slightly off the floor. Lower it again but don't let it touch the floor. Raise and lower it about ten times, keeping the leg off the floor the whole time. Keep the leg relaxed as you lift it. Imagine you are directing energy out through the kneecap to the side of the room. This image will ensure that the leg is always lengthening away from the hip, without tension, and not contracting back into the hip with the effort of lifting (fig. top left). Breathe out and in again naturally through the ten lifts.

* Breathe out and place the leg on the floor.

* Breathe in and repeat the ten lifts off the floor breathing naturally throughout, then breathe out and place the leg on the floor.

* Now take the right knee as far behind the body as is comfortable. Shift your weight forwards and support yourself on your hands on the floor in front.

* Breathe in and lift the right leg just off the floor. Raise and lower the leg behind you ten times, keeping the leg off the floor throughout. Try to maintain the image of directing energy out through the kneecap far behind you, and release any tension in the hip (fig. top right). Breathe naturally

Step 4 Strengthening

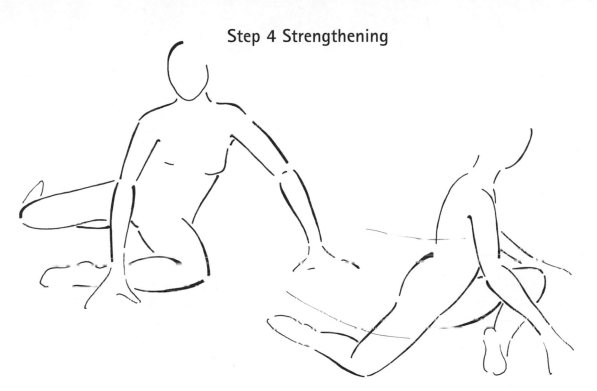

out and in again during the lifting.

* Breathe out and place the leg on the floor.

* Breathe in and repeat the ten lifts, then breathe out and place the leg on the floor.

* To come out of this, slide the knees to meet each other in front of the body then raise both knees so that you are sitting centre with knees bent and soles of the feet on the floor. Hug the knees to your chest a moment and breathe out any tension in the spine or hips.

* Elongate your spine, then begin again, this time by lowering the knees to the right side. Slide the left knee out so that it is pointing directly to the left side and the right knee is pointing directly in front of you. Release the hips and the shoulders. Shift your weight onto your right side and right hand and begin the lifts with the left leg. Do two lots of ten lifts to the side, then take the left leg behind the body and repeat the lifts.

* Come out of this as before by hugging your knees to your chest and curving your spine over the knees for a moment. Breathe out and release any tension before moving on to your next exercise.

*12 PELVIC TILT

This exercise strengthens the hips, bottom and the front and back thigh muscles.

Preparation

* Kneel on the floor on your mat or towel and sit back on your heels, with your spine long and upright and your hands placed in your lap.
* Breathe and relax the shoulder, neck and thigh muscles. Try to relax in this position, but if it feels uncomfortable, begin the exercise halfway through from the point of kneeling upright.

Sequence

* With a very slow, steady 'out' breath, curl your pelvis under, allowing your spine to curve a little. Keeping your pelvis curled under, raise up as slowly as you can to a kneeling position. At the same time, slowly raise both arms in front of you to shoulder height and, as you arrive in the kneeling position, open them out to the sides. Send energy out through the outstretched arms and use this image to raise the body. Release your pelvis so that you are kneeling up with a straight spine.
* Breathe in and relax.
* With a slow steady 'out' breath, reverse the movement. Begin by curling your pelvis under, curving the spine a little and slowly lowering towards your heels. At the same time, bring the arms together in front of you, reaching and sending energy out through the arms (fig. right). Keep your pelvis curled under until you are sitting back on your heels.
* Breathe in, straighten your spine, bring your arms down to your lap and relax.
* Try the raising and lowering movement ten times.

Notes

* The raising movement should feel like an opening and the lowering movement like a gathering in and enclosing. Try to join the movements together fluidly. Aim for a continuous movement coordinated with the slow breath.

Thigh Stretch, Step 5 (page 128) would be a good exercise to move on to after this one.

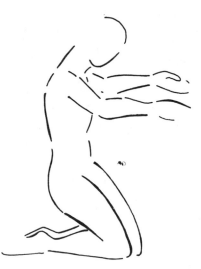

*13 GLUTEUS MAXIMUS

This is a specific exercise for toning the Gluteus maximus muscles of the bottom and thigh muscles and strengthening the small of the back. Some people may find the position a little uncomfortable and it is therefore best practised on an exercise mat or carpet. If you still find this exercise too uncomfortable, then use the All Fours Leg Lifts exercise (page 107), which works the same muscle group.

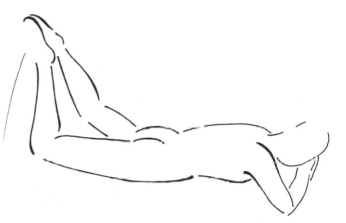

Preparation

* Lie face down on the floor on your mat or towel. Fold your hands under your head and rest your forehead or chin on them. Try to make your upper body feel relaxed and comfortable. Lift both feet up bending the knees so the legs form a right angle, and open your knees as far as is comfortably possible. Let the feet drop together to touch in the middle.

* During this exercise, imagine there is a piece of string attached to your toes and that it continues directly up above you. If the string is pulled upwards your legs and feet will lift as one. Concentrate on keeping the upper body relaxed throughout.

* Over a count of four, breathe in to prepare, elongating the spine and neck.

Sequence

* Breathe out over four counts and lift your toes to the ceiling. Send the breath and energy out through the legs and toes and directly up into the universe. The legs will not lift very high off the floor (fig. above). Imagine the energy as water flowing through your body. Be careful not to tense your body with the effort. If you find this movement difficult, try using the image of the string to pull your legs upwards by the toes until you can feel the sensations and muscle groups involved. Later, you can move to the image of the outward-flowing water energy to lift your legs.

* Breathe in and lower the legs carefully. Relax. As you breathe in air or energy, imagine that you are drawing it into your back and into the muscles that you have just been using, expanding them and creating space.

* Repeat the lifting and lowering ten times.

* To come out of this exercise, roll onto your right side and curl up, curving your spine around your knees. Slowly roll onto your back keeping your legs up by your chest. Hug the knees to the chest for a moment to release the muscles you have been using.

STEP 5

STRETCHING

1 ALL FOURS CURVE AND STRETCH

This very gentle spine stretch and whole body relaxation is a good one to use to finish off your daily exercise session.

Preparation

* Get down on the floor and kneel on all fours on your mat or towel. Place your hands directly in line with your shoulders and your knees under your hips. Leaving your back where it is, slide your hands out in front so that they are just beyond your head. Keep your spine very long and keep your head and neck as natural extensions of the spine.

Sequence

* Breathe in and curve the middle of your back up towards the ceiling as much as possible. Your head will naturally curve forwards a little towards your chest. Leaving your hands exactly where they are, slowly sit back so that you come to rest on your heels. Your arms and shoulders will stretch out (fig. below).

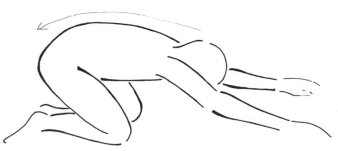

* Breathe out and release into this position. Feel the spine stretch as it curves over your thighs, and let your head and neck relax, dropping your forehead towards the floor. Feel the weight of the body pressing on the thighs. Release the leg muscles and let them succumb to the weight. Release your ankles and feet and release the shoulder joints. Breathe for a moment in this position, releasing a little more with each 'out' breath.

* Take a long energetic 'in' breath and use the breath to fill the body and lift it up, curving the middle of your back up to the ceiling until you are back in the all fours position.

* Breathe out along the length of the spine, elongating and straightening it, and return to the starting position. Begin again.

* Try the whole sequence three times. The exercise should be a very pleasurable release and relaxation.

2 SPINE BREATHING

This exercise relaxes the body, realigning the vertebrae and balancing the energy before you return to your everyday life. Here, it is performed on the floor with the soles of the feet together. If this position feels difficult or uncomfortable, the exercise can also be done sitting cross-legged, kneeling and sitting back on the heels or, most comfortably, sitting on the edge of a chair with the feet firmly on the floor in front of you.

Preparation

* Sit on the floor on your mat or towel, with the soles of the feet together and a comfortable distance away from the body so that the base of your spine is upright. Check that your spine is directly in the centre of your hips and sitting bones and that you are not pushing forwards or slumping back. Adjust your sitting position, if necessary, so that the spine is free to be straight. Place your hands lightly on your legs or in your lap if you are in sitting in another position, and relax your arms and shoulders.

* Breathe gently for a moment and imagine drawing energy into your body from the earth as you breathe in. Let it fill and lift your spine, fill your head, neck and face and create a sense of expansion and of space within. As you breathe out, allow the energy to recede back into the earth, leaving through the base of your spine.

* Feel a relinquishing of tension as the energy flows out. Let this image be gentle, like the ebb and flow of a wave. When you have this sensation clearly, increase the inward and outward flow of energy and integrate the body into the movement as follows.

Sequence

* As you breathe out, allow your head to curl down towards your chest, tilt your pelvis under slightly and let your spine curve from the base as much as possible (fig. top right). Use the relaxed weight of the body to deepen the curve. Release your hips. Consciously send the energy out through your body into the earth and momentarily

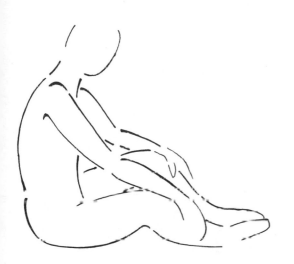

feel the sensation of being empty.

* Take a very drawn-out 'in' breath and allow the strong inward flow of energy to lift the spine, starting from the base. Let it fill the spine vertebra by vertebra, lifting your upper body up out of the hips, straightening your spine, lifting and opening your chest, filling your neck and head so that they rise up tall, and then escaping through the crown of the head.

* Let the 'out' breath begin almost imperceptibly from this lifted position so that the energy begins to recede from the base of the spine into the earth. Then send the energy firmly out and curve the spine over as before. Relax.

* Take about 10 – 12 'in' and 'out' breaths, using this spinal movement.

Notes

* If this movement and breathing cycle feels a little too fast for you to be able to work thoroughly with the spine, then extend it as follows: breathe in and rise up, then in the lifted position breathe out and relax the shoulders, breathe in again in preparation for curving the spine over. Breathe out and let the energy and breath recede down through the spine and into the earth, curving the back and tilting the pelvis under. Now, in this curved position, breathe in and then out and begin again.

3 CROSSED LEG STRETCH

A gentle stretch for the waist, the lower back and the muscles of the bottom and hips.

Preparation

* Sit on the floor on your mat or towel, with your legs crossed, arms relaxed and hands resting gently on your thighs. Sit up with your spine very tall, and breathe for a moment using the image of the Energy Fountain (see page 13), drawing energy in from deep within the earth and up through the base of the spine. Allow the energy to infuse and fill the body, creating space. Imagine some of the energy as water or light cascading down your face, shoulders, chest and arms then back into the earth.

* Be aware of which leg is crossed on top. Place your left arm across your lap. Breathe in and lift your right arm to the side and then up, as if tracing an arc on the far wall. When the arm is next to your ear, release any tension in the raised shoulder and then begin.

Sequence

* On the 'out' breath, lift up and over to the left side. Keep the waist long and take four or five small bounces over to the side, keeping your body and head facing front (fig. below).

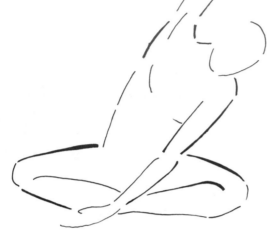

If you find you need support, place your left hand gently on the floor by your side.

* Breathe in and continue to bounce and reach over to the side for a further count of four or five.
* Breathe out and, in a fluid motion, slowly turn your body and head to face your left knee. Keep your arm raised up by the side of your head. Do four or five small bounces over your knee, reaching out with your arm to the left corner of the room. Keep your spine long and send the energy out through the raised hand, way beyond the body (fig. right).

* Breathe in and repeat the bounces, using the 'in' breath to lengthen and expand the body and elongate the reach.
* Breathe out and curve your upper body over your left knee. Relax.
* Breathe in, letting the air uncurl and inflate your spine until you are sitting centre and upright.
* Breathe out and release the shoulders, ready to begin again to the other side.
* Repeat the whole sequence to the other side. When you have finished, gently lift your knees, uncross your legs then cross them again, placing the other leg on top.
* Repeat the whole exercise, first with the right and then the left arm. Switching the leg position alters the stretch in the hip socket. You may notice that one side is much stiffer than the other. If this is the case, just observe this, be gentle and do not try to push it.
* To come out of this exercise, gently uncross the legs and shake them out until they are straight out in front of you.

4 UPPER BACK BREATHING

A gentle releasing exercise that focuses on the upper back and neck.

Preparation

* Lie flat on the floor on your mat or towel, with your arms by your sides, knees bent and soles of the feet flat on the floor. Lift your arms up wide to the side, just skimming the floor, and carry them on up behind your head. Bend your arms and place your hands behind your head. Throughout the exercise imagine you are sending energy out in front of you through the points of the elbows. This will help you sustain the lift without tension.

Sequence

* Breathe in and curl your upper body off the floor as far as the middle back or as far as you can comfortably, but keep your lower back on the floor. Curve your head towards your knees, reaching forwards with the elbows (fig. below).

* Breathe out and lower your spine one vertebra. Continue reaching forwards through the elbows. Imagine the 'out' breath is releasing the muscles of the back.

* Breathe in and stay at the same height. As you breathe, expand the lungs and the back outwards, to the sides. Feel your ribcage moving on the floor to accommodate the incoming air.

* Breathe out and lower one vertebra, still reaching forwards with the elbows.

* Breathe in, expanding the lungs to the sides and staying at the same height.

* Slowly work your way down the upper spine, lowering one vertebra with each 'out' breath, until the head returns to the floor. Try the whole exercise twice.

Notes

* As you do this exercise, try to notice the areas where you are stiff. Once you are aware of any stiffness, focus your Mind's Eye on those areas, breathe into them and begin to dissipate the tension. If you find one section that is particularly stiff, stay breathing at that point for two or three 'out' breaths until you feel some relief, then continue on up the spine. You could also try the Unblocking Energy exercise (page 149) from Chapter 3.

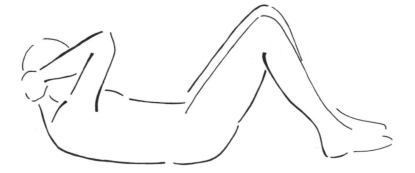

5 BACK ALIGNMENT

A very gentle exercise for releasing the neck and spine and for correcting the alignment of the back.

Preparation

* Sit on the floor on your mat or towel, with your knees bent in front of you and feet flat on the floor at a comfortable distance away from your body. Using your hands for support, slowly roll your spine down to the floor, gently pulling away from the hips and elongating the spine as much as possible until you are lying flat. Check that your neck is long, that your chin is not tucked in and that your jaw is released. Feel the whole back in contact with the floor. Breathe for a moment allowing your body to succumb to gravity.
* This exercise comprises three slow arm movements, each starting from and returning to the same position. The aim of the exercise is to focus on the sensations in the muscles and spine while moving slowly between the three positions. Lift your arms up directly above you towards the ceiling, tips of the fingers pointing towards each other, about three or four inches (7.5–10cm) apart. Your arms, chest and hands will form a long oval. Imagine that the oval contains light, energy, air, or simply a colour, and that you are containing it within your arms. This is your starting position.

Sequence

* The first movement stretches the oval upwards. Keeping the fingertips the same distance apart, slowly reach upwards with the backs of your hands as high as you can. As you reach upwards with your hands, allow your shoulders and then your shoulder blades to lift off the floor until only the centre of your back is in contact with the floor (fig. below). When you are reaching

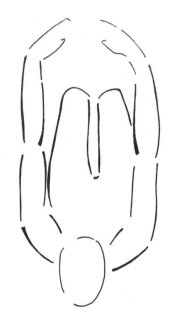

as high as you can, very slowly begin to lower your hands and upper body back to the starting position so that your hands are above your chest. Control the lowering of the hands and feel the shoulders and shoulder blades placing themselves on the floor. Try not to readjust the shoulders as they make contact the floor, but just let them lie as they are.
* The second movement squeezes the oval. Be aware of containing energy within your

arms. Keeping your fingertips the same distance apart, slowly lower your fingers towards the centre of your chest. Let your elbows bend, and imagine they are being pulled wide to each side. Feel your shoulder blades and your back muscles spread out across the floor. Squeeze the energy to your chest and finish with your fingertips just above the centre of your chest. The arms should be off the floor. Breathe for a moment and feel the sideways movement of the ribcage on the floor as you expand your lungs. Slowly raise your hands back to the starting position and, as you do so, be aware of the movement of the shoulders on the floor. Check that there is no tension in the front of the neck or the shoulders or in the legs or feet. Your arms will be beginning to feel quite heavy now. Simply be aware of this.

* The third movement opens out and releases the oval. From the starting position, very slowly start to move your fingertips away from each other, as if you were freeing the substance that you have been carrying and letting it dissipate into the atmosphere. Control the slow movement of the arms as they open out and travel down to each side, and send energy out through the arms to each side throughout. When your arms are about three or four inches (7.5–10cm) off the floor, hold them in this position and breathe. As before, be aware of the muscles in the back in contact with the floor. Feel the weight of the arms and feel them tingling as you send energy out through them (fig. below). Slowly begin to raise the arms, bringing them together again. They will feel very heavy. Imagine that you are drawing the energy from your energy field back into you and are slowly enclosing it in the oval as you return to the starting position. Once your hands are above your chest again, breathe and relax.

* Try the whole three-movement sequence three times. Breathe naturally throughout the exercise. Aim to join all the movements together so that the exercise flows without pausing.

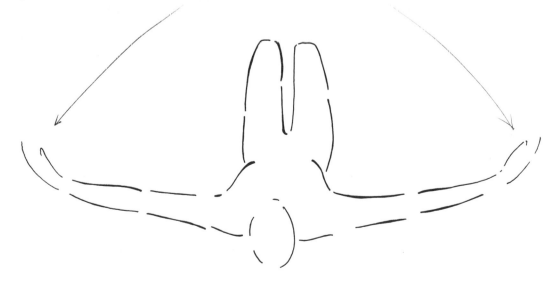

6 DIAGONAL SHOULDER STRETCH

A stretch for the shoulder joints and upper back.

Preparation

* Lie flat on the floor on your mat or towel, with your knees bent in front, soles of the feet flat on the floor, and your arms relaxed by your sides.
* Breathe for a moment and concentrate on elongating your spine and the neck. Feel the whole back in contact with the floor.

Sequence

* Breathe in and reach diagonally across your body with your right hand to the outside of the left knee, lifting your right shoulder and upper back as far off the floor as you can.
* Take hold of the outside of the left knee. Breathe out and relax, and stretch the shoulder joint while holding onto the knee.
* Bend your left arm and take hold of the right arm by the wrist. Release the knee, and with the left arm, pull diagonally away from the knee, elongating the right arm and shoulder (fig. top). At the same time, slowly lower your right shoulder back to the floor, using each 'out' breath to release the shoulder a little more.
* Place your right arm back down by your side, and begin on the other side by reaching diagonally with the left arm across to the outside of the right knee and lifting

your left shoulder and upper back off the floor. Proceed as before.
* Try the whole exercise twice on each side.

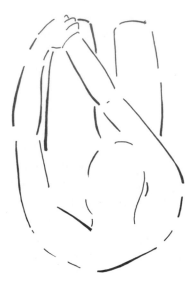

7 HIP STRETCH

An exercise that alternately stretches and strengthens the very powerful muscles of the hips, bottom and the top of the thighs.

Preparation

* Lie on the floor on your mat or towel, with your knees bent, soles of the feet flat on the floor and your arms relaxed by your sides. Be aware of the whole of your back in contact with the floor.
* Lift your right knee up towards your chest and rest the right ankle on the left thigh, letting the right knee drop to the side as far as is comfortable. Breathe in and lift your head and upper body just enough off the floor so that you can join your hands around the back of the left thigh. To do this, you will need to thread your right arm through your legs.

Sequence

* Use a very long, drawn-out 'out' breath to gently draw your left thigh towards your chest, leaving your right leg exactly where it was placed and placing your shoulders and head back on the floor. You will feel a stretch in the muscles in the right hip and bottom. Use the 'out' breath to dissipate the stiffness (fig. top).
* Breathe in and relax. Release the pull from the arms, but keep your hands around your thigh.
* Using a long drawn-out 'out' breath, press away from the body with the right leg against your left thigh. Keep holding your

left thigh as before. This is an isometric movement, and you will not move very far. Allow your head and shoulders to lift off the floor slightly and to be elongated by the stretch. The hand hold and the contrary pressing with the right leg strengthen the muscles of the right hip (fig. below).

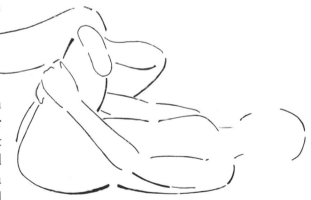

* Breathe in, release the press and relax.
* Use the 'out' breath to gently draw the left leg towards the chest as before. Continue alternating the drawing towards you and the pressing away, and try four of each in total.
* Slowly release the left leg and lower the

foot to the floor, then place the right leg on the floor.

* Repeat the exercise on the other leg. Begin by raising your left knee towards your chest. Place the left ankle across the right thigh. Let the left knee drop to the side and relax the leg. Breathe in and place your hands around your right thigh, threading your left hand between your legs and lifting your head and shoulders slightly off the floor. Continue as before, gently pulling your right leg towards you with an 'out' breath, then releasing and relaxing with an 'in' breath. On the next 'out' breath, press away from the body with the left leg. Breathe in, release the press and relax. Again, try four in total.

8 THIGH STRETCH

This stretches the fronts of the thighs and hips.

Preparation

* Kneel on the floor on your mat or towel and sit back on your heels. Breathe for a moment, elongating the spine, and letting your shoulders drop away from the neck and your arms hang by your sides.
* Place your palms on the floor slightly behind you and walk them back behind you a couple of steps until you are leaning right back away from your legs. Support the weight of the body on your hands. Make sure your head is not jutting forwards but that it is in a straight line with your spine.

Sequence

* Breathe out, lift your bottom up slightly from your heels and press upwards with your hips for a count of ten (fig. below).

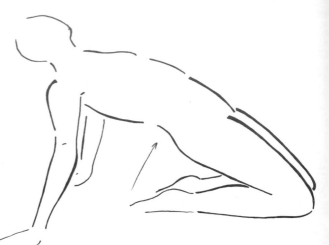

* Breathe in, release the upward press and slowly lower your bottom so that you are once more sitting on your heels.
* Repeat the upward press once more, and release back down to the floor.
* Now breathe out and lift up slightly from your heels. This time press only one hip up for four or five counts, then change and press the other hip high for four or five counts, feeling the lengthening in the front of the thigh and hip.
* Breathe in and repeat the four or five count upward press with the right and then the left hip.
* Breathe naturally and slowly lower to sit back on your heels. Walk your arms and body back to the upright postion. With a firm 'out' breath release any tension in your legs and shoulders.
* Try the whole sequence twice in total.

*9 WAVE STRETCH

This is one of my favourite whole body stretches that feels so good to do, a little bit like a cat stretch. The stretch moves in a continuous wave, and it may take a few tries for you to get the coordination right.

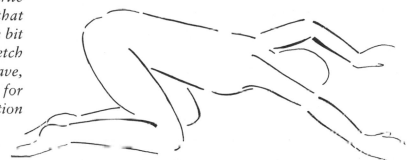

Preparation

* Kneel on the floor on your mat or towel and sit on your heels. Don't worry if this feels a little uncomfortable, since you won't be staying in this position for long.
* Place your hands lightly on your thighs. As you breathe for a moment, elongate the spine and allow the shoulders to drop away from the neck. Release the top of the thigh muscles and relax the ankles if possible. Simply allow the legs to be folded and feel the weight of the body pressing through them.

hands, bending your arms and pass your chest as close to the floor as possible. You will feel as if your bottom is left stuck up in the air momentarily (fig. above).
* With the 'in' breath continue travelling forwards, chest leading the way. Slowly push up through your arms and straighten them. Your legs will straighten automatically. As you push up through your arms, reach upwards with your chest towards the ceiling, and let your stomach and legs touch the floor (fig. below).

Sequence

* Breathe out and begin the wave by curling your head down towards your chest. Continue to curve your spine over towards your knees, reach out and place your hands in front of you on the floor. Now move forwards, taking your weight onto your

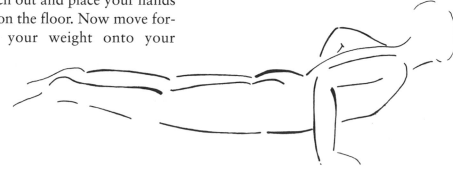

Allow the head to tilt back slightly as a natural extension of the spine and the upward opening of the chest. This is the end of the first part of the wave (fig. right).

* Breathe out and reverse the wave by trying to retrace the path that you followed. The reverse wave is led by the hips. Feel

them pulling the body back. Let the chest remain upwards for as long as possible, then bend the arms and pass your chest very close to the floor.

* Begin the 'in' breath as you feel the weight of the body transfer onto your knees. As your hips pull you back to the original kneeling position, keep your chest as close to the floor and then as close to the knees as possible. Once you are sitting on your heels, let the 'in' breath inflate and uncurl your spine, vertebra by vertebra, so that the head uncurls to upright last of all. Arms relaxed by your sides.

* Breathe out, allowing your shoulders to drop and relax and letting the thigh muscles release with the weight of the body. Feel your spine long and straight before you begin the whole sequence again.

* Try at least three complete wave stretches continuously, or do as many as you enjoy.

Notes

* Once you become familiar with the pattern of movement and the sensation of the different parts of the body leading, try to focus on the continuous wave-like motion of the body. Imagine you are part of the falling and receding of the waves on the shore line. The water moves through you and you are carried forwards with the force of the sea. In the same way as with Wave Breathing (see page 15), try to let the movement flow without stopping so that the turnaround movement is part of the natural flow. Even the pauses to breathe between waves can become fluid and part of the wave.

*10 OVER THE TOP SPINE RELEASE

This is a powerful spine release using the breath. There are many variations on this stretch, but this version is the most basic for releasing and stretching the spine. This exercise should be approached very gently.

Once you are familiar with it, experiment with and adapt it according to what feels best for your spine. If you have any problems with your spine, avoid this exercise completely. For reasons of comfort it is best to remove any hair clasps or necklaces and avoid wearing a ponytail, since these may cause discomfort during the exercise. You will definitely need a mat or towel for this exercise.

Preparation

* Sit on the floor on your mat or towel with your knees bent in front of you, feet parallel and flat on the floor. Curl your spine down vertebra by vertebra, elongating the spine away from the hips, until you are lying on your back. Place your arms by your sides.

Sequence

* With an 'in' breath, swing your bent legs up and over your head. If you find this difficult, place your hands in the small of your back to support you. Your knees will end up above your forehead or, if you are very supple, on either side of your head by your ears. Breathe several times, releasing into the stretch with each 'out' breath.

* Now work your way down the spine, vertebra by vertebra, using the breath to release the spine as follows. Breathe in and fill the spine with the breath, then as you breathe out allow the spine and legs to move down about one vertebra. Feel the weight of the body spread through that vertebra and let it release and open. Leave the

legs naturally bent and keep them as close to your chest as possible. The challenge here is to keep your balance. The relaxed weight of the legs will help you balance in the position. If this is not enough, place your arms over your ankles and use their additional relaxed weight to counterbalance you. If this is still difficult, place your hands in the small of your back for support.

* Stay in this position. Breathe in and let the breath fill the spine and spread through the muscles of the back, creating space and light in the muscles and vertebra.

* Breathe out firmly and roll down one vertebra. Send the 'out' breath, along with the stiffness and toxins, firmly out through the spine and also through the legs (fig. below).

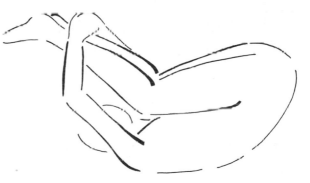

* Continue in this way, breathing and opening the back, vertebra by vertebra, until you reach the small of the back. Carry your bent legs on down and place your feet on the floor. Relax.

* It should be sufficient to do this exercise once only, although if you do it twice, the muscles of the back will feel much softer and the spine more open the second time.

* To come out of this stretch, roll onto your right side and curl up. With your back still curved over, roll onto your knees. From the kneeling position, slowly uncurl the spine with an 'in' breath before standing up.

Notes

* If you sense a dull stiffness in any one particular part of your back, then adapt the exercise accordingly. Just stay and breathe in and out through the same vertebra two or three times until you can feel it opening and clearing, then continue down the spine. If your whole spine feels very stiff, try rolling down the whole length of your spine with one long 'out' breath. Do not focus on any one vertebra, but massage all of them with the rolling action. Then place your feet on the floor. Swing your legs up and over again with an 'in' breath and roll all the way down the spine again with one long 'out' breath. Keep the legs as close to your chest as possible until the very last moment.
* If this exercise is uncomfortable for you, use the Upper Back Breathing (page 123) or Back Alignment (page 124) exercises. In addition, use the Curl Down exercise (page 35) from Step 1 to release the spine. After several months of exercising and moving the spine, you can try returning to this exercise.

*11 SPIRAL STRETCH

A strenuous spine, shoulder and hip stretch. Do not use this stretch if you have any problems with your spine. Instead use one of the gentler stretches such as All Fours Curve and Stretch (page 119).

Preparation

* Lie flat on your back on the floor on your mat or towel, with your legs outstretched and your spine and neck long. Extend your arms out on the floor, level with your shoulders.
* Breathe for a moment, filling the body through the five points as you breathe in through both arms, both feet and through your head. Breathe out firmly through all five points, elongating all the limbs and releasing the muscles.

Sequence

* Bend your right knee and lift it up towards your chest. Carry the knee over to the left side, allowing the body to roll slightly to the left and letting the lower spine come off the floor. Try as much as possible to leave both arms stretched out on the floor where they are. The spine should form a spiral from the hips up to the shoulders, with your head and neck lying flat. Unless you are very supple and can take the knee all the way down, hold your right knee off the floor, with the calf and foot simply hanging relaxed below the knee (fig. right).
* With a slow, firm 'out' breath, send energy out through the extended right arm. At the same time use the 'out' breath to release the right leg and allow the weight of the leg to lower it a little towards the floor. Send energy out directly to the side through the bent knee. You should be able to feel a connected line of energy spiralling through the body from the right arm across and out through the right knee.

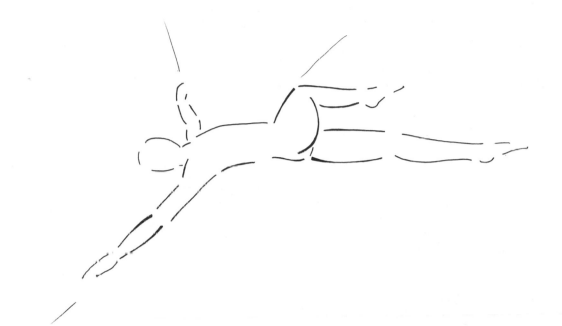

* Breathe in and fill and elongate the spine with the breath, leaving the leg where it is, then breathe out and release into the stretch as before, breathing out through the right knee to the left side and reaching way across the floor with the right arm in the opposite direction. Try this four times in total.

* To come out of this, slowly raise the right knee and allow your spine to roll back straight so that it is flat on the floor. Once the spine is straight, place your right foot on the floor and slide the leg down to join the left. Breathe for a moment through all five points, elongating the spine and the limbs.

* Repeat the stretch with the left leg. Begin by bending the left knee and lifting it towards your chest. Carry the leg over to the right side, allowing the spine to spiral. Keep the arms and shoulders reaching wide to the sides. As you breathe out, send the breath firmly out through the left arm, release the left hip and allow the weight of the leg to lower it a little to the floor. Feel a direct line of energy spiralling through the body from the left arm and shoulder to the left knee and beyond. Continue as before.

Notes

* Focus in this stretch on the energy images and the direction of the breath. See the 'in' breath clearing a space in the muscles of the back, shoulders and hips, drawing in replenishing energy and light. Breathe out firmly and dispel all the used energy and waste from the muscles completely through the five points of the body.

*12 DIAGONAL REACH

An energetic stretch involving the whole body.

Preparation

* Stand in the centre of your exercise space and spread your feet wide apart to the sides. Raise your arms wide to the sides at shoulder height. Breathe and feel how your body is very open in the centre. Imagine you are sending out energy through the five points. Breathe in to start.

Sequence

* Breathe out and bend your right knee deeply. Holding your shoulders and arms in the same relationship to each other, spiral in the waist so that the left arm swings forwards and the right arm swings back and the shoulders are facing the right side. Now lean forwards over your right knee and touch your left hand to your right foot. The right arm should be pointing directly up into the air. Your head will naturally turn to the right. If you can, turn your head to look up along your right arm to increase the stretch (fig. right).

* Breathe in and raise the body up to face front again and straighten your legs. Keep the arms spread wide to either side.

* Breathe out and bend deeply on the left leg. Spiral in the waist so that the right arm swings forwards and the left arm back, and your shoulders and head turn to face the left side. Now lean forwards and touch the left foot with the right hand, with your left

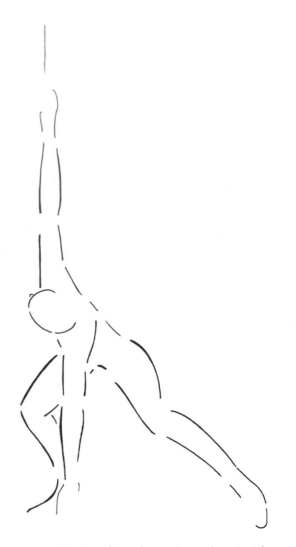

arm pointing directly up into the air. If you can, turn your head to look up along the raised left arm.

* Breathe in and raise the body up to face front, straightening the legs.

* Try ten in total, alternating right and left. Finish with the right hand touching the left foot.

* To come out of this exercise, bend and slowly lower the left arm, bend both knees and bring your body to the centre, curved

over between your bent legs. Let your shoulders, arms, neck and head hang down between your legs for a moment. With a firm 'out' breath, release any tension. Breathe naturally. In your own time, breathe in and slowly uncurl your spine and straighten your legs until you are standing upright.

Notes

* Try to develop your own rhythm that coordinates the breath and the movement confidently. The movement with the 'out' breath should feel like a dive as you push into the floor with the legs, taking the body over and your arm down to the foot. Begin with steady controlled movements. If you speed up the rhythm later, do not swing wildly, but control the bending and the spiral and carry the arms. The faster the rhythm, the greater the strength that is required in the centre of the body to control the weight of the arms and the swing.

*13 CHAIR STRETCH

An intense stretch for the legs, hips and upper body. You will need a chair for this exercise. The higher the chair, the more intense the stretch.

Preparation

* Stand in front of the chair so that the chair back is furthest away from you. Lift your arms up wide to the sides just below shoulder height and send the energy out through them to the sides. Raise your right leg, straighten it and place the foot on the seat of the chair. Check that your supporting leg is directly underneath you. If it is not, adjust your distance from the chair. Relax the raised leg and imagine it is very long.

Sequence

* Breathe out and bend the left leg, keeping the foot relaxed on the floor and keeping your spine upright. Keep the raised leg straight throughout the first part of the exercise.
* Breathe in and use the breath to straighten the left leg and lengthen the spine.
* Repeat the bending and straightening once more.
* Now breathe out and bend the left leg as before and reach your arms and upper body over the raised leg towards the chair back. Take hold of the chair back if possible, the right leg remains straight throughout.
* Breathe in and, leaving your back where it is, straighten the left leg. At the same time, use the breath to elongate the spine and the raised leg (fig. overleaf).
* Repeat the bending and straightening once more, keeping your back in the same position.
* Now breathe in and bend your right leg, placing the sole of the foot flat on the chair so that it can take some of your weight.

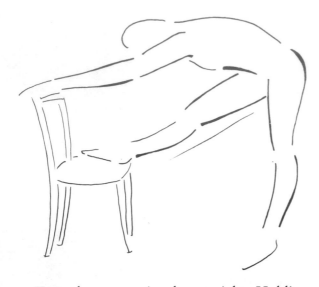

Keep the supporting leg straight. Holding on to the chair back for support, draw your hips and body gently towards the chair. You will feel a stretch in the front of the left hip and calf and the right hip and back of the thigh.

* Breathe out and slowly straighten the right leg. Leave your hands on the chair back and stretch out the spine and the arms and shoulders.

* Repeat the bending and straightening of the right leg once more.

* To come out of the stretch, bend your right leg slightly, curve your spine, lift the leg from the chair and place it on the floor.

* Now repeat the whole exercise, starting by raising the left foot in front of you onto the chair.

* Try the whole exercise four times, twice on the right and twice on the left, alternating legs.

Notes

* The exercise is made up of a pattern of six bendings and straightenings: two with the supporting leg only, two with the supporting leg and upper body reach, and two with the raised leg, in towards the chair.

* If you are particularly tall, once you are familiar with the exercise, you may want to try placing the leg on something a little higher like a chest of drawers or window ledge. I'm nearly six feet tall and my legs reach a window ledge without effort! The general rule is never to have the raised leg higher than the hip. At the maximum height, therefore, the raised leg would form a right angle to the supporting leg. Take care also to choose an object or piece of furniture that will not collapse or topple over under the weight of your leg and the pressure of the stretch.

TO FINISH...

WAVE BREATHING

This relaxation exercise from the Energy Fountain (page 13) is an excellent way to finish off your Daily Energy Exercises, if you have the time.

Preparation

* Stand with your feet parallel and as wide apart as your hips, arms by your sides.

Step 5 Stretching

Sequence

* As you breathe in, let your knees bend as deeply as they can, without raising your heels off the ground. At the same time, allow your arms gently to raise in front of you. Imagine your arms are resting on top of water so that they feel buoyant and supported from underneath without effort (fig. below).

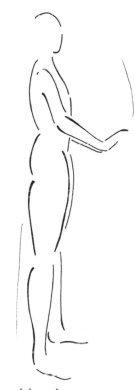

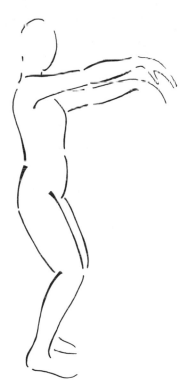

* As you breathe out, press the heel and palm of each hand down through the 'water' and at the same time straighten your legs. Feel a slight resistance as you lower the arms, as if pushing them against the water's surface (fig. top right).
* Continue the movements described above Try to find a natural rhythm that combines the breathing with the movement so that your arms and hands are an expression of the movement of the breath. Focus on the wave-like nature of the movement. There is no top or bottom to the wave, only continuous motion, and the breath is relaxed and easy, not forced. The turn-around moment of the wave – the ebb into the flow – is almost imperceptible. Allow the breath to move in the same way so that it is not held at the top or at the bottom, but a continuous wave.
* When you feel you have focused enough for today, come to stillness at the end of an 'out' breath. Stand still for a moment and take the opportunity to thank your body for its service to you.

DAILY ENERGY SELECTIONS

The following selections are intended to assist you with your initial choice of exercises, and all can be practised in a 20–30 minute session. Over time, you can add or eliminate exercises according to your individual preference. Don't forget to choose one or two exercises from the Energy Fountain to commence your daily session.

BALANCED DAILY ENERGY SELECTION
For an all-round exercise session

	Step
Upward Reach	1
Skiing Swing	1
Sitting Bounces	1
Concentric Circles	2
Arm Press	2
Flamenco Contract and Open	2
Leg Brushes	3
Outer or Inner Thigh Chair Press	3
Sitting Side Stretch	3
Cycling	4
Curl Up	4
Hip Stretch	5
Diagonal Reach	5

HIGH ENERGY SELECTION
For when you are feeling particularly energetic

	Step
Skiing Swing	1
Spiral Swing	1
Gathering and Opening	1
Drawing Energy	1
Side Stretch	2
Towel Stretch	2
Flex and Push	3
Figure of Eight	3
Travelling Knee Lifts	3
All Fours Leg Lifts	4
Swinging Your Weight or Twister	4
Wave Stretch	5
Diagonal Reach	5

REVITALIZING SELECTION
A great revitalizer if you are feeling rough

	Step
Upward Reach	1
Curl Down	1
Side Stretch	2
Shoulder Chair Stretch	2
Flex and Stretch	3
Sitting Side Stretch	3
All Fours Leg Lifts	4
Pelvic Push Up	4
Thigh Stretch	5
Wave Stretch	5
Over the Top Spine Release	5

Daily Energy Selections

RELAXING SELECTION
Releases tension, aids digestion and sleep

	Step
Swing, Bounce and Shift	1
Curl Down	1
Sitting Bounces	1
Toxin Release	2
Hand and Arm Circles	2
Heel Raisers or Front of Thigh	3
Leg Circles	4
All Fours Curve and Stretch	5
Spine Breathing	5
Back Alignment	5
Wave Breathing	Chapter 1

MINIMUM MAINTENANCE
My most frequently used exercises in a 20–30 minute session

	Step
Swing, Bounce and Shift	1
Upward Reach	1
Curl Down	1
Spiral Swing	1
Drawing Energy	1
Toxin Release	2
Side Stretch	2
Concentric Circles or Arm Press	2
Foot Strengthener	3
Leg Brushes	3
Front of Thigh	3
Outer Thigh Chair Press	3
Sitting Side Stretch	3
Spiral Slide	4
Cycling or Twister	4
Crossed Leg Stretch	5
Over the Top Spine Release	5

THE ENERGY SOURCE IN THE OFFICE

Many of the Daily Energy Exercises can easily be done in a break at work or even while you are sitting at a desk. If you are feeling tired or sluggish, just five minutes of exercise will refresh you. To do the exercises sitting at your desk, sit forwards on your chair with a very straight spine, lifting high out of the waist and hips. Release your chest, shoulders and arms and breathe for a moment, expanding the chest and ribs, before you start exercising. Place your feet flat on the floor in front of you and, if possible, slip off your shoes, so that you can feel the whole of each foot in contact with the floor.

Try The Energy Fountain preparatory exercise (page 13) to refresh you totally. This exercise can be done whilst sitting at any time without anyone else noticing. As you breathe, imagine that you are drawing breath and energy directly into your body through the base of the spine. Imagine a strong connection of energy through the spine to the earth. As in the original exercise, allow energy to pass through the body, creating space in the muscles and joints. Allow some energy to pass up the back of your neck, to circle inside your head and then travel beyond the body through the crown of the head. Let it cascade down around you, releasing your face, shoulders, chest and arms as it returns to the earth. Send it directly down into the ground through the base of the spine, as well as through the legs and feet.

The following exercises do not require much space and need no special preparation. Select according to the amount of time you have available.

	Step
Swing, Bounce and Shift	1
Curl Down	1
Toxin Release (can be done seated)	2
Side Stretch	2
Elbow Press (can be done seated)	2
Shoulder Chair Stretch	2
Foot Strengthener (can be done seated)	3
Flex and Push	3
Heel Raisers (use chair back)	3
Front of Thigh (use chair back)	3
Inner Thigh Chair Press (can be done seated *See P.143)	3
Cycling	4
Curl Up	4
All Fours Curve and Stretch	5
Spine Breathing (can be done seated)	5
Crossed Leg Stretch	5
The Energy Fountain (can be done seated)	Chapter 1

*To do the Inner Thigh Chair Press sit upright on your chair, rather than on the floor, make a loose fist with one hand and then place the fist, knuckles on top, between your knees. Follow the instructions for the original exercise (page 87), pressing your knees together onto the fist with the 'out' breath and releasing and relaxing with the 'in' breath.

THE ENERGY SOURCE FOR TRAVELLERS

When travelling you may find yourself in a confined space for long periods of time, for instance in an aeroplane, on a train, or in an airport lounge or a waiting room. All of the seated exercises for the office can be applied in these situations. Also, simple hand and foot circling will enliven your whole body. Travelling, particularly foreign travel, may involve many changes of food, time zones, sleep patterns and stress levels from trying to cope with a foreign climate or language. The impact of these can be minimized by continuing to exercise and listen to your body. Do not give up your routine and the time you put aside for yourself simply because you are in a strange environment. Your body will be trying to normalize itself and rid itself of extra toxins. 'Little and often' is the key. Even five minutes of stretching a day is worthwhile and preferable to abandoning your exercise session totally for a week or two. Although many hotel rooms are very cramped, you will find sufficient Daily Energy Exercises that do not reequire much room. Switch off the neon striplight and try to let in some natural light and, if possible, 'natural' air while you exercise. Place a towel on the floor. This delineates your exercise space and focuses your concentration. It also separates you from nylon carpets and any garish patterns! If there is anything inspirational to look at in the room or anything that you might have brought with you, have it within view. If not, try having a glass of mineral water near you. Sip it between exercises or drink it afterwards.

If you are very short of time, there are a couple of shortcuts that you can use. Upward Reach (page 32) can be done in the shower or while getting dressed; the Towel Stretch (page 69) can be done while drying off; the Foot Strengthener exercise (page 73) and Heel Raisers (page 77) can be done in front of the washbasin; Curl Up (page 102) can be done in the bath and Outer Thigh Chair Press (page 86) can be done against the sides of the bath while bathing.

If circumstances simply have not allowed you to maintain something of your exercise routine, be aware that after a couple of days absence from exercising, possibly combined with alcohol, added stress and poor eating habits, your muscles will be very stiff and full of toxins. Drink plenty of water and concentrate on the general clearing, breathing and stretching exercises. Try the suggested Revitalizing Selection. Be gentle and breathe through the stiffness. It usually takes the same number of days that you have abstained from exercising to return to your normal level of fitness, although you should feel immediate improvement within a day.

The Energy Source

The following exercises are very useful in a confined space such as a train corridor or small hotel room.

	Step
Swing, Bounce and Shift	1
Upward Reach	1
Curl Down	1
Knee Bends	1
Toxin Release	2
Side Stretch	2
Elbow Press	2
Arm Press	2
Towel Stretch (hotel room)	2
Foot Strengthener	3
Heel Raisers	3
Outer Thigh Chair Press (hotel room)	3
Inner Thigh Chair Press (hotel room/can be done seated)	3
Pelvic Push Up (hotel room)	4
Pelvic Lift (hotel room)	4
Spine Breathing (can be done seated)	5

CHAPTER 3

THE REMEDY

As you practise the exercises from the Energy Fountain and the Daily Energy Programme you will begin to feel the combination of the images and the breathing working on your overall sense of wellbeing. After a few weeks you may begin to notice that you are more relaxed and have a more positive outlook in general and that you feel 'lighter' on your feet. The Energy Source works at a very deep level in the body, not just by muscle-building and toning, but also by clearing and changing long-established energy patterns. It promotes deep relaxation and enables you to adopt new ways of moving and thinking about energy which can transform the body.

As you work with the three key elements of The Energy Source – Intention, Breathing and Listening in to the body – you can begin to apply these to your daily life and help prevent or help to alleviate the symptoms of many everyday stress-related problems. In this chapter are several simple techniques that can be practised in five or ten minutes during a break from work to refresh and release energy. These techniques use images and ideas that you have already encountered earlier in this book and apply them to specific symptoms. At the end of this chapter is a quick reference guide, outlining which techniques to use to help alleviate different symptoms. I have also included a few simple self-massage ideas which are marvellous for relieving tension in a short space of time.

BREATHING AND RELAXATION

Strong, full breathing is an essential element in The Energy Source work to encourage a clear flow of energy through the body and ensure efficient detoxification. Full breathing promotes a deep relaxation in the muscles, making them more efficient and improving the functioning of many of the internal organs. So many of us tend to breathe using only a fraction of the capacity of our lungs. Our breathing may also be constricted as a result of poor posture and physical health and, of course, our emotional state of mind.

Try to develop the habit of listening in to your breathing occasionally and become aware of how you breathe. Observe the rhythm of your breathing. Do you have a tendency to hold your breath slightly after the 'in' or 'out' breath? If so, when performing the exercises, try to release this hold and allow your chest to rise and fall in a continuous gentle motion. The turnaround point from the 'in' to the 'out' breath, and vice versa, should be almost imperceptible as in the Wave Breathing exercise (page 15). Which part of your lungs are you using predominantly?

When doing the exercises, consciously open the areas that you are not using, and allow the breath to expand them.

The following exercise encourages the lungs to be used to their full capacity. This exercise can also be used at any time to promote relaxation or to calm anxiety.

SIMPLE BREATHING EXERCISE

This exercise develops three distinct movements of the lungs: stomach breathing; back breathing; and upper chest breathing. It then combines them to create deep, confident breathing and relaxation.

* Lie flat on your back on the floor with your spine very long and your arms relaxed by your side. Bend your knees and place the soles of the feet flat on the floor. The whole of your back should be in contact with the floor. Breathe naturally for a moment and observe the breath. Is it calm, fast, shallow, agitated, constricted, deep, slow? Try to calm the breathing as you observe it.

Stomach breathing

* Now place your palms lightly on your stomach, just below your ribs. As you breathe in, consciously draw the breath down and imagine that it is filling the stomach. Imagine the air circling around as it expands your stomach.

* Now send the breath through your stomach and into the palms of your hands. Notice how your hands rise as the stomach fills. As you breathe out, gently press the air out with your hands. Take four or five deep breaths, filling the stomach and the palms of the hands. Breathe gently and do not force the breath.

Back breathing

* Next, place your hands on your ribs at the sides of your body. Take a deep breath in and imagine the air circling in the rib cavity and creating space. Send the breath beyond the ribs into the palms of your hands. Expand the lungs and ribs out to the sides and use the breath to actually push your hands away to the sides. Feel the breath filling your back and feel your ribs and the shoulder blades moving across the floor to accommodate the breath.

* As you breathe out, gently press the air out with your hands. Be aware of the ribs moving against the floor to return. Take four or five deep breaths, expanding the lungs to the sides and sending the breath into the palms of your hands.

Upper chest breathing

* Place your hands on your upper chest. Breathe naturally for a moment and soften any gripping in your chest and shoulders. Imagine that as you breathe you are able to send the air through your chest and into the palms of your hands. This creates space in the chest and dissipates any tightness.

* Breathe in deeply and now deliberately fill the upper chest with the breath. Notice how your hands rise as the air circles and expands the front of the shoulders and chest. Feel the weight and the warmth of your own hands.

* As you breathe out, press down gently with the hands and send the air out. Take four or five deep breaths, filling the upper chest and passing air through the chest into the hands.

Now connect all three movements in one long 'in' breath. Continue to place your hands on the different areas if you need to to check that you are really filling them.

* Draw the breath in and send it into the stomach, then let it rise, circling to expand the ribs to the sides, then softening and expanding the upper chest as it fills the whole body cavity.

* With one long 'out' breath reverse the order. Send the air out of the upper chest, bring the ribs in and press down gently on the stomach until the lungs are totally empty.

* Begin again immediately. Take four or five long breaths, focusing on filling all three areas fluidly.

As this exercise generates a lot of energy and increased oxygen flow, you may find yourself a little dizzy momentarily. When you have completed the exercise, relax for a moment on your back and allow your breathing to return to normal before you get up.

If you find one of the three areas particularly constricted or difficult to isolate, then concentrate for a while on that one area. To release the constriction, add the following variation to the simple breathing exercise.

Simple Breathing Exercise Variation

*Go into the breathing exercise as described above, concentrating on your chosen area.

* Focus your Mind's Eye on the rise and fall

of the breath as before and try to imagine the air, light and energy circling in the body, creating wonderful space. Be aware of the warmth that is coming from your own hands, as you breathe into the palms.

* Continue breathing and very slowly take your hands about an inch (2.5cm) away from the surface of your body. Imagine that you are still sending the breath beyond the body into your hands. Let the surface of the body soften and expand to allow the breath to pass through it and beyond.

* After a while, slowly take the hands a little further away with each 'in' breath. Eventually remove the hands completely and breathe for a moment as if they were still in place. The area should have released a lot of its tension and your breathing should be much easier.

BELLY BREATHING

This exercise promotes deep relaxation, aids the functioning of the digestive system and internal organs and is also effective in removing stomach or period cramps. It is particularly beneficial if you do it while you are lying in bed, just before you go to sleep.

* Lie flat on your back with a very long spine and neck. Bend your knees and place the soles of your feet on the floor. If you are in bed, place a pillow under your knees and totally relax the legs, allowing them to go very heavy. Breathe naturally for a moment and calm your breathing right down over four or five breaths.

* Place the palms of your hands lightly on either side of your belly or lower abdomen, then relax your arms and elbows down by your sides so that you feel the weight of your hands on your belly.

* On an 'in' breath draw the air right down through your body and expand your abdomen with the breath. Observe your belly and hands rising as you fill the area. Imagine that you are drawing in so much air that you can see it circling around your abdomen, creating space and dissipating any tension. Feel the warmth and the energy passing from your hands into the belly. Now send the air out beyond your abdomen and into your hands. Imagine the hands lifting and opening away from the body as if to accommodate this generous expansion.

* Breathe out and send some of the air down through your belly into the legs and out of the body via the feet. Send some of the air firmly out through the lungs and also out through the top of the head. This should feel like a wonderful clearing away of tension and toxins. Imagine them being washed away with each ebb and flow of the breath.

* With each 'in' breath soften and open the abdomen more, and with each 'out' breath experience a relinquishing of stagnant energy and a creation of space and relaxation in the body.

* Take at least five deep 'in' and 'out' breaths, preferably more, until you feel deeply relaxed. As you do the exercise, try to take your Mind's Eye down into your abdomen, and focus only on the rise and fall of the breath and on filling the hands.

* To finish, very slowly raise your palms about one inch (2.5cm) from your belly. Continue to breathe and now send the breath beyond the surface of your body into the palms. Feel your belly soften and expand as the breath passes through it and beyond. Experiment a little. With each 'in' breath, slowly take the hands a little further away from the belly, eventually up to about 12 inches (30cm) away. Notice how long you can feel a connection between the palms, the stomach and the breath and at what distance you lose that connection. Slowly remove your hands completely and breathe for a moment as if they were still in place.

UNBLOCKING ENERGY

This is a technique for releasing stiffness and unnecessary holding in the body that can block the free flow of energy. If left unchecked, it can lead to tension headaches, stomach cramps, digestive problems and tight muscles. Ideally, as you become more aware of your body and get into the habit of listening in, you will be able to release the energy blocks before the symptoms completely manifest themselves. However, the following unblocking method can also be used to relieve symptoms should they occur.

Alternatively try it at the end of the Energy Fountain exercises just to check into the body and monitor how you are doing.

* If you have just completed the Energy Fountain preparatory exercises come to a relaxed standing position. If you are using this technique on its own, stand with your feet as wide apart as your hips and for a moment just become aware of your breathing. Over four or five breaths, calm the rhythm of the breathing, concentrating on breathing out and emptying the lungs completely each time. With one firm 'out' breath, release your shoulders and chest and let your arms hang by your sides.

* Now as you breathe, cast your Mind's Eye through your body and see if you can identify the source of the tension or holding. Where is it located? You may notice several areas. Focus on the one that seems the strongest. The most common areas for blocked energy are the shoulders and neck, the stomach and diaphragm, the small of the back, the front of the chest, or the back of the head, the jaw and temples. Try to identify your own areas as they may well be more specific and subtle than this. As you look with your Mind's Eye, the kind of sensations that you might encounter are that the area is solid and not free-flowing, or it may be denser than the rest of the body or very dark. Alternatively, you may experience it more as a physical sensation. The area may feel crunched up or knotted, or there may be a dull ache in it. Any of these signals will do.

* Decide which sensation is most prominent and then take one hand and place it as best you can over that area. Leave the hand in place and then consciously relax the arm and shoulder. Breathe. Begin to be aware of the hand touching the body, feel the weight

of the hand, then the warmth passing from your hand into the body. Draw the breath into the body, using the image of the Energy Fountain. See the breath circling throughout the body, and direct it into the blocked area. Breathe into the tension and through it and beyond, into the palm of your hand. After several deep breaths, you will begin to feel the area expand and lighten. Imagine that the breath dissipates the block as you breathe in and then expels the resulting toxins from the body as you breathe out.

* Once you begin to experience a lightening and relinquishing, gently lift your hand away to about an inch (2.5cm) from the body. Continue to breathe through the block and into the hand and feel the area open more as you raise the hand. Very slowly draw the hand away from the body, breathing all the while, and replace it by your side. Continue to breathe through the area for a moment as if your hand were still in place, recalling the sensations.

* If you have time, take your Mind's Eye back into the body and identify the area that now gives the strongest signals. Then work on that block in exactly the same manner. Repeat the whole sequence as often as you like with other areas. If you are generally tired and you experience many areas as dull, try the same technique but with the hands placed lightly over the eye sockets or on the scalp. This is very soothing and relaxing and seems to open the whole body.

This exercise is wonderful done with a partner. It helps develop a trust and a sensitivity between two people.

To do this, cast your Mind's Eye through your own body as before and then indicate to your partner the area that needs releasing. Your partner should rub their hands together vigorously first to generate some warmth, then place a hand on the area while you relax. Be aware of the warmth and the weight coming from your partner's hand. Then concentrate on breathing into the hand and dissipating the tensions. After a while your partner should gently lift their hand away as described in the unblocking method above, while you continue to breathe into it as if it were still in place. Alternate roles so that each of you has the opportunity to release the other's energy blocks.

TENSION HEADACHES

Tension headaches can be eased and often removed completely by using the unblocking method described in the previous exercise. If you feel one coming on and are able to take five minutes to do something to dissipate it, try the following exercise.

* Sit on a chair, keeping a long straight spine and neck. Place your feet flat on the floor in front of you. Release your shoulders and arms and place your hands, palms upwards, in your lap. Breathe for a moment, using the Energy Fountain image. Imagine drawing the light or water energy up through the floor into your feet and also directly into the base of your spine through

the chair. Imagine it flowing into your shoulders, under the shoulder blades, up the back of your neck and up into your scalp behind the ears. Feel these areas expand and lighten as the energy circles through them. Draw the breath in and send it into these areas and then out beyond the surface of your body into your energy field. Breathe out, sending the air and spent energy through the crown of your head and down through your body, back into the earth. Clear the lungs and the body completely, making way for the next inrush of fresh, light energy or water.

* As you feel the tightness begin to ease a little, place your hands lightly over the temples, on the scalp or over the eye sockets, depending on where the centre of tension is located. If you are unsure, use all three positions one after another in this order. Use the unblocking method of breathing into the palms. Imagine also the warmth of the palms having the power to melt the tension away.

* Sit and breathe until the area begins to clear a little. Gently take your hands off the surface of the skin about one inch (2.5cm) and continue the breathing for a moment. As the area relinquishes its tension, move on and focus on the next area.

* To finish, slowly lower the arms and replace them palm upwards in your lap. Sit quietly for a moment until the calm in your head has established itself before continuing with your day.

THROWING THE BREATH

A very simple and yet effective movement for ridding the body of negativity and stagnant energy. This movement is best done after massaging or unblocking energy or after the Daily Energy Exercises as a kind of finishing off.

* Stand in the centre of your space, facing a window or facing outdoors so that you have some sense of a distant horizon. Take a strong, active stance with the legs, for example have one leg forwards, one leg back and your knees bent. You are going to use your arms to describe the drawing up of energy from the earth, through the feet and up into the body as you breathe in deeply.

* Keeping your feet and legs firmly planted on the floor, throw your arms and upper body towards the horizon, hurling the 'out' breath and any unwanted energy and negativity as far away as you can with your arms. Keep your body, arms and hands totally relaxed, like a rag doll. Repeat this three or four times until you feel lighter. If you have no window in your space, hurl the energy and breath down into the floor some way in front of you.

THROWING YOUR WORRIES

This is a simple but effective way of ridding the body of persistent and unwanted thoughts and mental chatter. It can be used at the beginning of the Energy Fountain preparatory exercises or before the Daily Energy Exercises if you are having trouble concentrating. It can also, of course, be used completely on its own as a quick method of relieving anxiety.

* Stand with your feet as wide apart as your hips. Unlock the knees and for a moment be conscious of the rise and fall of your breathing. Continue breathing naturally and calmly and stand very still.
* Now take your awareness into your mind and become aware of all the movement that is going on there. For now, simply observe the thoughts going round and round as if in a washing machine. Continue breathing steadily. Begin to identify the different thoughts that are present. Pick them out – 'I haven't done such and such'; 'I haven't got time to be doing this'; that horrible newspaper image that won't leave you; or what so and so said to you about your work, and so on. You obviously have your own dialogue. Pull them out one by one and imagine that you could catch them in your hands until you have them all there in front of you, jabbering away simultaneously. Stifle their chatter by closing your hands.
* Now begin to knead them together into a tight compact dark ball. Really wring them out and squash them in your hands until they hold together in a solid ball and their individual voices are just a blur. Take the ball in one hand, take a deep 'in' breath in preparation and now breathe out and hurl the ball as far as you can into the horizon. Watch it go. Hear the blurry voices recede until they disappear totally. Sense the lightness and clarity in your head. Now you are ready to gently begin your exercises or to return to work.

BODY VIBRATION

A simple device for shifting blocked energy, revitalizing and encouraging the free flow of energy.

* Stand in the centre of your space with your feet as wide apart as your hips, arms relaxed by your sides and shoulders and chest relaxed.
* Keeping the whole body relaxed and fluid, begin a small vibration in the lower part of the legs. Focus on keeping the vibration as regular and as small as possible. Now make the vibration travel up your legs and, as it does so, try to release the thigh muscles to the vibration. Carry the vibration on up the body. Try to feel it in the small of the back, then release the back and shoulder muscles to the vibration. If you can, soften the front of the chest and allow that to vibrate and, finally, involve the head and the face. See the vibration passing from the crown of your head into your energy field.

152

* Keep the movement going until you can feel the large muscle masses of the body letting go. Then release the movement and shake out the energy from the limbs and the body into the floor.

MASSAGE

Massage is a very good technique for deeply relaxing the body, breaking down stubborn fat deposits and encouraging a healthy elimination of waste and toxins. Although traditionally we might think of massage as some form of indulgent treat performed by a specialist, there are many ways in which we can benefit our wellbeing with a few moments of easy self-massage. The following four massages are the simplest and most effective to perform on yourself and have all the benefits of a massage given by someone else.

If you suffer from diabetes, epilepsy, high blood pressure, eczema or other skin complaints, or if you have any bone or ligament problems or are pregnant, do not attempt any form of self-massage. If in doubt, consult your doctor. Use the other remedial techniques for breathing and unblocking energy to rid the body of tension.

VIGOROUS ENERGY RUB

This is a very easy method of revitalizing the energy in the body if you feel sluggish. It can be done before your Daily Exercise Programme or at any other time on its own.

* Stand relaxed and begin by circling and rubbing your palms together until you start to generate some warmth.
* With one hand, begin at the base of the neck, on the opposite shoulder. Squeeze the area firmly with the whole hand, hold the squeeze for a moment and then release it. Work your way down the shoulder, upper arm, elbow, forearm, wrist, hand and fingers, squeezing firmly, holding and then releasing the area. Work as if you were moving the tension along down the arm and out through the fingers, as if you could wring it out like squeezing a tube of toothpaste. Lastly, take a firm hold of the fingers being massaged and draw your working hand down so that you elongate the hand and fingers. Shake the working hand out, directing the tension and spent energy into the earth.
* Repeat the squeezing movements with the other hand, starting at the base of the neck, on the opposite shoulder.
* Now, using the palms of your hands begin to make large, vigorous circles over your chest, then over your stomach, and then move around to the small of your back and down over your bottom. Now make the circles smaller and faster as you work your way down both thighs and calves. Bend your knees and curve and relax your

back over as in the Curl Down exercise, so that you are not creating any additional tension. Keep your arms relaxed as they work, focusing on their easy, circular movements and not on any effort involved. As you reach the feet, stroke your hands firmly over the length of the feet, from the ankles to the toes, and onto the floor. Shake out your arms and fingers, directing the tension into the floor. Repeat the foot stroke and shaking movement a couple of times, or as often as you like. You should now be feeling a lot warmer and revitalized.

FOOT MASSAGE

According to oriental medicine, the feet are key massage points, with different areas of the feet corresponding to and stimulating different vital organs and body functions. You will certainly find that a simple foot massage will enliven your whole body and circulation and promote a general sense of wellbeing. The following massage is particularly beneficial if used prior to commencing the preparatory Energy Fountain exercises, as it increases your awareness and receptivity and opens the body to an increased energy flow.

* Sit comfortably on the floor, with your legs relaxed and bent in front of you. Make sure the feet are warm – you could wear socks if you like. You are going to do the whole massage first with one foot and then move on and repeat it with the other foot.

To begin, rub the palms of your hands together vigorously to generate some warmth, and then hold the foot to be massaged between both hands, with one palm on the top of the foot and the other palm against the sole. Feel the warmth of the hands for a moment and then begin to rub the foot by circling the hands.

* Starting with the little toe, work your way through all the toes, circling them each in turn. Take hold of the little toe between your thumb and first finger. Make four or five circles in one direction and then four or five circles in the opposite direction. Then move on to the next toe and repeat the circles and so on for all five toes.

* Now, take hold of all the toes firmly with one hand and, squeezing tightly, draw the hand down the length of the toes, elongating the toes. As your hand releases, shake out the tension from the hand into the floor. Do this squeezing and drawing movement two or three times or as many times as feels pleasurable.

* Using the heel of one hand press and stroke into the sole of the foot. Make a firm long stroke from the heel to the toes. As the sole of the foot is quite delicate, you may find certain areas tender. Try to use an even pressure with the hand rather than pressing the fingers into the tender areas. Repeat this stroke four or five times.

* Moving on to the heel of the foot, cup the heel with the whole of one hand and firmly rotate the fleshy ball of the heel in one direction for four or five rotations, then in the the other direction for four or five rotations.

* Take hold of the whole foot and, using

your hands, make four or five circles with the foot around the ankle joint. Keep the foot and ankle relaxed and let your hands take the weight of the foot and do the circling.

* Using your fingers, make small circles, massaging around the bones of the ankle and the Achilles tendon at the back of the heel. Use a constant but gentle pressure as the bones here are small and complex.

* With the edge of the thumb, continue the gentle pressure down the top of the foot towards the toes. Work with the thumb between the tendons on top of the foot, ending up by pressing between the toes and drawing the thumb out between the toes and away beyond the foot. Work with the thumb from the ankle in this way down and away between each of the toes, so four strokes in total.

* To finish, use the palm of the hand to stroke the top of the foot from the ankle to the toes and away to the floor. Do this several times, shaking the hand out and sending any tension into the floor at the end of each stroke.

* Now move on to the other foot and repeat all of the above. If you're not already wearing one, put a sock onto the foot that you have just finished working on so that it does not get cold.

FACE MASSAGE

A face massage is very simple to perform and can easily be done in a five-minute break from work. The face, particularly the jaw, often carries large amounts of emotional tension. You will find that this brief massage brings relief from tension and refreshes you.

* It's best to perform this massage from a sitting position, although it can be done standing. Before you begin, breathe for a moment, consciously drawing the breath up into your head and neck. See the breath circling inside the head and creating space. Imagine the breath filling the back of your neck, moving up behind the ears then across the scalp and down across your face. Send the breath out firmly through your mouth and also up the back of your neck and out through the crown of the head.

* Take the index fingers of both hands and press them on either side of the bridge of the nose. Now pressing gently, trace the line of the eyebrows out to the temples. Release the pressure a little each time you pass over the temples as these are delicate areas. Still using your index fingers, start again from the bridge of the nose and this time trace a line a little higher up the forehead, parallel to the eyebrows. Maintain a constant pressure with the fingertips until you reach the temples, and keep the movement smooth. Repeat this movement four or five times, each time tracing the line a little higher up the forehead parallel to the eyebrows. The last movement should trace

a line along the hairline and out to the temples. Finally, use both hands to smooth and stroke the whole forehead from the centre to the temples.

* Place both index fingers on either side of the bridge of the nose again and exert a gentle pressure either side of the bridge by pressing the fingers towards each other. Next, slide both fingertips up so that they are pressing up into the browbone. Now slide the fingers outwards, following the line underneath the eyebrows, gently pressing into the browbone.

* From the bridge of the nose again, you are going to press down the sides of the nose and then out along the edge of the cheekbones, underneath the eyes and out towards the temples. Be very careful not to press into the eyes, only onto the bones. This time press a point and release it, move along the cheekbones, press and release again so that you are pressing a series of points along the bones rather than making one long continuous movement out to the temples.

* Now use the edge of the index fingers to trace a line from the bridge of the nose all the way down the sides of the nose. Pause and increase the pressure a little at the bottom of the nose, pressing under and into the nostrils. Repeat this a couple of times.

* Still using the edge of the fingers, press firmly and trace the line from the edges of the nose to the corners of the mouth.

* Now start in the centre of the chin. Take hold of it between the thumb and bent index finger of both hands, thumbs under the jaw, fingers on top. Squeeze firmly and follow the jawline out to the left and right towards the ears. Squeeze and release then move on, squeeze and release again and move on, taking about four moves to reach the ears.

* Place your fingers on your cheeks, just in front of the ears, and find the muscle that joins the upper and lower jaw. With the first three fingers of each hand, exert a constant pressure on the muscle for a few moments. As you hold the press, breathe into the jaw muscle and imagine dissipating the tension with the breath. Breathe the toxins out firmly, releasing the jaw area. Repeat this movement with the muscle on the lower jaw.

* Take hold of the earlobes between the thumb and first finger of each hand. Press them and draw the fingers down, until the earlobes are released. Repeat this movement a couple of times.

* To finish, close your eyes and place the palms of your hands lightly over both eye sockets and sit calmly for a moment. Breathe and draw the breath into your head. See it circling in a light, clear cavity in your head and up the back of the neck. Imagine you could breathe through the eyes and send the breath beyond them into the palms of the hands. Relax the eyes in their sockets. As you breathe, be aware of the warmth of your hands. When you feel relaxed and refreshed, slowly remove the hands and continue breathing through the eyes for a moment. Open your eyes, and you are ready to return to your work.

HAND MASSAGE

Sit in a comfortable position for this massage. Ideally, rub some hand cream or moisturizer into your hands before you start, although the massage can also be done without. You are going to work one hand first and then the other. Try to keep the hand that is doing the work as fluid and relaxed as possible and keep the working shoulder released.

* Begin by generally kneading and squeezing one hand with the other, paying particular attention to the heel of the hand, the knuckles and the fingers.

* Now take hold of the hand to be massaged by placing the working thumb on the palm and the index finger on the back of the hand. Pressing the thumb and index finger together, work your way down the back of the hand towards the fingers, between the tendons. End each stroke by squeezing the fleshy part of the hand between each finger. Take four moves to work your way across the back of the hand, starting between the thumb and first finger and working across between each finger to the little finger.

* Using the working thumb and index finger, take hold of the little finger at the base. Squeeze and circle all the way down the finger, giving an extra squeeze at the very tip before releasing the finger. Work your way down from the base of each finger, squeezing and circling, finishing with the thumb.

* Massage the fleshy base of the thumb on the heel of the hand. Now take hold of the flesh between the base of the thumb and first finger and press for a moment then release. As you press, use the working thumb on the palm side and the index finger on the back of the hand. Hold the press long enough to imagine drawing the breath into the hand and dissipating the tension beneath your fingers. Breathe the tension out firmly and relax your hand. Rub the area gently after the press to release any remaining tension.

* Using the working thumb flat against the palm, begin on the heel of the hand below the thumb joint and make a firm steady stroke upwards towards the fingers. Repeat this movement working across the heel of the hand and palm in four strokes, finishing each stroke at the base of the fingers.

* Massage, working in gentle circles around the wrist bone, using the thumb and first two fingers.

* To finish, take hold of the whole hand again. Squeeze and press it, moving from the heel of the hand down the palm. Take hold of the fingers firmly and draw them out long, sliding the working hand down the fingers until you must finally release them. As you release the tip of the middle finger, shake out the tension from the working hand into the floor.

* Begin again and repeat all of the above with the other hand.

QUICK REMEDIAL REFERENCE

SYMPTOM	SUGGESTED METHOD
General tension. For a five-minute break at work.	Face Massage Hand Massage, Belly Breathing Body Vibration, Throwing the Breath
Anxiety/stress	Simple Breathing Exercise Throwing Your worries Throwing the breath
Tension headache	Unblocking Energy Face Massage
Poor digestion	Belly Breathing
Stomach cramps	Belly Breathing
Period cramps	Belly Breathing
PMS	Daily Energy Programme
Sleeplessnes	Daily Energy 'Relaxation' Selection Belly Breathing
General stiffness	Unblocking Energy Daily Energy 'Revitalizing' Selection Vigorous Energy Rub
Low energy	Vigorous Energy Rub Foot Massage, Body Vibration Daily Energy 'Revitalizing' Selection

The above can be used to alleviate the on-coming stress-related symptoms of occasional complaints. If your symptoms are regular, persistent or severe consult your doctor immediately. You may be able to continue to use the Energy Source remedial methods to complement your treatment, but ask your doctors advice before continuing.

CHAPTER 4

THE ADDICTIVE DANCE

Dance was my first love and most probably will remain my last. It has been my greatest teacher, holding the strings to the obsession that undermined my health and reduced me to a very bleak point in my life, yet conversely it has also held the key to my healing.

I started dancing at the age of two, too early to say that I had consciously chosen it for myself as a way of life. I recall early on that my dancing brought pleasure to my mother who at that time was recovering from cancer and suffering from overdoses of radiation. I had the sensation that my dancing was somehow inextricably linked with her survival and life force, a fairly powerful message for one so young. I continued and excelled. By the age of seven, I was training as a classical ballet dancer three or four hours a day, despite regular school work. By that age I was hooked, not by the vision of me as some sylph in a white tutu, but by the struggle against my own body to achieve beauty and perfection and for the moments of near transportation that attaining that perfection brought. I was lifted out of normal life by focusing on the line of the body, the rhythm, the music, the connection I felt to the movement and to the energy. To train and constantly push past the limits of physical endurance too, had its own kind of high, now acknowledged and understood amongst athletes. As I reached my teens, experts started to say I was gifted but that I would never make a dancer because I was too tall. This was another challenge to rise to. 'I'll show them,' I thought. I ignored my gifts in other areas such as mathematics and sciences – these came too easily to me for my liking! I committed my life to dance and to the beginning of my journey. Dance was almost like a religion to me. The concentration and focus necessary to achieve what was required of the body was all-consuming. The training required such intense focus that you could literally become 'one' with the movement as you worked. You could lose all sense of 'self' or being bound within a limited body and become one with the flow of energy.

As I trained, I began to realize that rather than abandoning myself to this sense of 'oneness' and the energy, I could in fact harness it and use it to my own ends to intensify and improve my performance. For example; if I focused on increasing the energy flow at a certain moment, I could jump and be suspended in the air for what seemed like forever. In a balance 'en pointe', on the toes of one foot, with the other leg raised high, I could stay there for what seemed an unnatural amount of time if I directed the energy flow downwards, firmly into the earth, to act as roots. Yet this was the very opposite of what we were encouraged to think of in order to balance. This ability to harness the energy extended the near ecstatic moments in which I felt beyond physical limitation. Yet, for dancers, hand in hand with this striving for perfection of sensation and movement, goes an unprecedented determination, armour-plating and self-denial. The most destructive and self-defeating of these is the denial of personal comforts and denial of sustenance and food. As a result, many dancers live with debilitating illnesses such as anorexia and bulimia. Pain and suffering are also denied as part of this fight for control and perfection. I recall at the age of 11 being encouraged to put neat surgical spirits on open cuts on my feet to try and toughen them up. My feet were always a mass of weeping blisters, cuts and swellings, which I simply had to ignore. The denial of energy levels, illness and injury is quite phenomenal. As a teenager I danced with a temperature of 104, determined not to be stopped because I was sure that I was simply being weak and sure that I could conquer it. We danced and trained whatever.

Although I did not really appreciate it at the time, I was very fortunate that, unlike most of my contemporaries at the residential ballet school I ultimately attended, I did A-levels and studied music as well. I continued to train for the same three or four hours of ballet a day as I had done at regular school, while most of the other pupils trained in classical ballet seven hours a day. I noted then that there was a limit to the extent that you could train a body without the mind and spirit being exercised in balance. I appeared to progress further than the other students on half the amount of training because I was able to maintain a sense of perspective and balance the physical training with other mental stimulation. Dancers tend to spend so much time focused on themselves physically, regarding the body as an instrument to be trained, that they can emerge with a lack of balance in life. They usually have very little sense of self or self-worth, since a dancer is totally dependent on the praise of others. This is how we are trained. We hang on to every criticism, every compliment, every review, to try to get a sense of what is real and what works. Any other sense of self is given away to the dreaded mirror. Every move is assessed first by the mirror image, rarely from within. We are never enough. We constantly strive to jump higher, turn faster, be longer, thinner, taller, never giving ourselves the satisfaction of being okay as we are. As a result, a constant self-deprecating inner dialogue becomes a way of life, only to be exacerbated later by the competition and constant rejection as we enter the world of work.

Making a living out of dance comes as a short, sharp shock that few dancers are ever prepared for. Young hopeful dancers will do almost anything for the future possibility of dancing in a respectable company or show. They traipse off to clubs and cabaret contracts all over the world in the hope of putting together their six months provisional Equity requirement. I led something of a dual life. I was studying music and dance at London University, and yet at a phone call from the Parisian entrepreneur I worked for, I would drop my studies and fly off to France or Italy or Cairo to do a cabaret for him. The money and lifestyle was very attractive to one so impoverished in London. Somehow I was able to overlook the seamier side of it. It all seemed surreal to me, since in 'real' life I was a student.

At the age of 20, as the end of my degree loomed, a mixture of pride and desperation attracted me to accept a 14-month contract for MGM in Las Vegas as a showgirl, earning more than I've ever earned since from dance. It took about a month for the glamour of the star-studded show and the novelty of the lifestyle to wear off. When I managed to escape my contract and regain a sense of what was important to me in life, I began to view myself as a 'serious' intellectual dancer, which meant doing things for the love of it because it had artistic integrity. The only way I could support myself financially in this contemporary dance career was by working as a fashion model. Working on a cat-walk was actually a lot easier on my spirit than dancing in a cabaret. At least I did not feel I was prostituting my art. Unfortunately, this situation did not last for ever and so I decided to make my living doing only what I loved – dancing in serious works for choreographers that I respected.

One of the turning points for me in my 'serious' contemporary dance career was auditioning for a famous and well-respected choregrapher in Germany. All the dancers had travelled a long way to dance for her in good faith. For the first several hours of the gruelling audition she was not in attendance. When she arrived she seated herself in front of the mirror with her back to us and viewed us all indirectly via our mirror image, whispering and joking continuously with a colleague. Later when she needed to communicate with us, she would not look anyone in the eye, even though she was addressing us directly.

She set a series of movement combinations which were to be done partnered by one of the other auditioning dancers. The combination began slowly and increased in speed as it repeated itself. She told us she would say stop at a certain point. To do this combination actually involved inflicting pain on one another. Both partners tried very hard of course, as they wanted to please, but as the speed increased, she omitted to say stop. She simply watched to see what we would do and at what point we would give up. My sense of self-worth finally reared at this treatment and I stopped, much to the dismay of my partner. Ultimately, when the last stragglers had come to a standstill, to add insult to injury, she indicated vaguely in our general direction and said she wasn't looking for any dancers anyway! I felt so angry on behalf of all of us who were trying so hard to please and who were dancing for the love of it.

I continued to perform for people I respected and began creating my own choreography, but from that point on I began to question. The first thing that concerned me was the unspoken 'no pain, no gain' maxim of the daily training. It seemed to me that if I trained only when it felt right to do so, when I was really focused and concentrating, it was bound to produce better results than if I forced myself to train when I did not want to. Equally, I began to question whether I should perform things in the name of art that felt harmful and were against my own better judgement.

This attitude was viewed almost as heresy and seemed to challenge others in the profession. As I began to choreograph for myself and others, I became more sensitive to how different we all were and realized that the way to encourage someone to give their best was to listen to their body and to them and to work with their individuality. The idea of listening to and nurturing the individual was very much contrary to the prevailing artistic aesthetic, and it took a long time before I was actually able to implement these ideas successfully in my own life.

In order to survive, I began working seven days a week, five of which were spent teaching professional contemporary dance in London, with one day teaching in the north of England, and one day as the rehearsal director, choreographer and performer with a new company. By this time I knew I had a grumbling foot injury, which was very inconvenient, so I ignored it. I found that by shifting my weight and not landing correctly when performing jumps, I could work around it for a while! After six months without respite on this gruelling routine, I was totally drained. In an attempt to compensate for my foot injury, I had injured other joints and now had an injury that was screaming for attention. I had to stop.

With the help of a very supportive friend, I was able to begin my search for practical ways of healing my foot injury. The initial advice I received was to do absolutely no physical exercise at all for about three months. According to the doctors, my joints were like those of a 60-year-old. 'Joints only have a finite life,' I was told. 'Use them up and they're finished.' At this point in my life I had been dancing for nearly 26 years, so to do nothing was a pretty drastic move for my body. The joints of the 60-year-old very soon took over and manifested themselves throughout my body. I totally seized up. The joints seemed to solidify to such an extent, that whenever

I sat down, I had difficulty getting up again and would be stuck in whatever position I had got myself into. Besides which, my foot injury was as excruciatingly painful as ever. I had to do something, so I decided to try an alternative medical approach to my injury.

The first practitioner I saw came up with the prognosis that I obviously subconsciously did not love my left foot enough! It may well have been true, but I was not ready to listen to anything like that. The next alternative practitioner concluded by asking if I'd had a traumatic birth. I told him that as it happens I did, but I was really looking for a more practical solution so that I could get on with my life. By this point, I'd undergone a series of X-rays and knew that one of the supporting bones under my foot had at some point during my performing split into two and now functioned as two completely separate free-floating pieces of bone. As a result, I soon found myself before a leading orthopaedic surgeon at a London hospital.

I was examined by a group of nervous students that he had brought along with him. Very shakily one volunteer student tested the mobility of my hip joints and monitored my leg movement. With a few helpful hints about angles and hand holds from me, we successfully managed to test my hip flexor muscles. The other students stood by and took copious notes because the joints were hypermobile and way beyond anything they had come across in a textbook. After about half an hour, I told them this was all very well but that the trouble was in my left foot and could they take a look at that. 'You see, students, what did I tell you,' the surgeon said. 'Always listen to the patient.' With a quick cursory glance at my foot, he announced: 'Oh that's very simple, we'll just remove the bones.' Somewhat aghast, I asked him what he would replace them with. 'Nothing. Why?' came the reply. 'Why!' I said. 'Because these are supporting bones of my foot, and if you simply remove them without replacing them, it's going to shift my spine and my alignment about a centimetre.' He told me it was a very simple operation and that he did it every day of the week. 'That may well be the case, but I only have one left foot and I'd prefer to keep the bones even as they are,' I replied. 'I give you four weeks,' he said. 'You'll change your mind.' He parted with a flourish, leaving me alone in the cubicle wondering where to turn next.

My first thought was that I simply had to move and exercise in some way. Doing nothing was only making matters worse. What did normal people do? Something like a Jane Fonda workout, I suppose. I had never done anything like that before. Full of a renewed sense of positivism I set off to get myself a workout video. I found my workout video truly awful, so fast, punishing and unrelenting. I was shocked. Could people who hadn't trained every day for more than 26 years really do this stuff? I couldn't. There was absolutely no way I could do all the repetitions required of me. I couldn't keep up. I persisted, humiliated that I was obviously so out of shape. After about a week of this exercise I was feeling pretty stiff. As I sat in a chair, trying to recover from that morning's workout, my back very slowly began to slump over towards my knees. I tried to relax. I was obviously tired, I told myself. The whole process of deterioration took about a half an hour. I could not lift my back upright from its collapsed position.

There was an osteopath located just around the corner, and I decided I had better take myself off to his office at once. Stubborn and determined as ever, I levered myself from the chair bent double. I called a friend and told him I was in a bit of a fix, then with the help of my arms, which thankfully still seemed to be working, I began to claw my way down the stairs and out to the garden wall. As I attempted to cross the drive, dragging my legs behind me, I realized this was not going to work. It it had taken me half an hour to get this far. Perhaps the osteopath could make a house call? On the way back upstairs I made it about halfway and gave up. Dramatically strewn across the landing, unable to continue, was where my friend found me. The osteopath arrived, and I was carried upstairs and laid on my side on the bedroom floor, where it transpires I was to stay for the next five days. The osteopath said that he could not get near me I was in such spasm. So long as I didn't move, I wasn't in any pain, so there I stayed.

Prior to this, I had agreed to make a guest appearance with the contemporary dance company I had helped form, to dance a piece that had been specially created for me. At the time, I had thought it a crazy idea, given my injuries, but had decided to do it anyway. I crawled to the phone on hands and knees to tell the company of my sorry predicament. They didn't believe me and put the composer, a close friend of mine, on the phone. Wasn't this excuse a bit elaborate, he asked. Why didn't I just admit that I didn't want to do the performance? Initially I was annoyed that he thought I'd go to such lengths to get out of dancing. Later, when I reflected, it seemed in truth, that I'd had to create a scenario in which I was not able to walk before I could let myself off dancing. I had a doctor visit me to check that I had not damaged any nerves. Fortunately, I had not. The osteopath also called several times but said that he could see nothing wrong and could do nothing for me. Was this it, I wondered as I lay there? Had I lost all my fight? My friends were very good for me, making me laugh as I crawled my way about the flat. One day, as they were about to go off on a river boat party, they cracked jokes about taking me along on a stretcher. They left laughing. I heard their laughter trail off down the hallway and into the car. I was alone.

I stared at the ceiling. How long could I go on lying here? Until I decided I wanted to be well and would listen to myself and be gentle and kind, came the answer. Not really knowing what I was doing, I rolled onto my side and levered myself up onto my feet. I was a pretty poor specimen, bent over at 90 degrees and twisted, but at least I was standing. With the help of the wall, I began to walk slowly. Taking very shaky paces at first, I managed to walk the length of the wall. I turned round and made my way back in the other direction. I thought of nothing except breathing and the will to walk. I walked and I walked, probably for near on four hours, although I was not very conscious of time. As I breathed through my spine, it slowly began to straighten without pain until, finally, I was tentatively upright. I had been longing for a bath, so I very gingerly lowered myself in one, determined that when my friends returned I would be standing upright, dressed, clean and wearing make-up.

As I sat in the bath, a series of wonderful healing images came to me, of walking in the Sierra mountains and high desert, of cross-country skiing frozen landscapes and cycling free against the wind. A whole pageant of joyous activities, the likes of which I had never even entertained before in my life, came into my mind. I vowed that I would open my eyes and start to appreciate the world beyond the ballet studio. I would be walking, cycling and skiing into my old age. Some hours later, my friends burst through the door, scanning the floor to tell me what fun they had had. They stopped short. Their faces and their silence at seeing me are an image I shall not easily forget.

This was the turning point. From then on I looked to myself for healing and for the answer on how to restore both my mental and physical health. I decided that the solution was to keep moving, as I had 'walked' that day. Ignoring the doctors, I started to move in a gentle way every day. I worked with what I knew, easing and coaxing my joints into mobility, breathing and releasing my muscles, relinquishing old-established patterns of tension and effort. I drew into my body a lightness and gentleness that were totally new to me. I followed my own wisdom, and my body responded rapidly.

What began to emerge from my daily explorations was a series of gentle exercises that I could draw on. I explored the nature of breathing and its fundamental relationship to my body and to movement, something I had never done before. I realized that energy and movement were united by the breathing. I felt the connection between breathing and a strong energy and life force. I looked at the quality and flow of energy through my body and the effects of my thought patterns on that energy and my body's response. I listened to my body attentively, constantly monitoring its responses and trying to answer them. On a more practical level, I developed movements with shapes and patterns that were beautiful and satisfying to do and looked for ways of gently strengthening the body that required no effort. In essence, I tried to involve my whole being and whole consciousness into the process of my healing.

From that point on, life took me into to many new and unexpected areas. By this time, I desperately needed to earn some money, but what on earth could I do? I had spent my life inside the four walls of a studio, before a mirror, working with my body. I considered the question that if I couldn't dance, what else had ever given me joy? I had a recollection of a single moment, dancing for Opera North, an opera company based in northern England, where I had been surrounded by about 50 wonderful singers all breathing and singing into my body. Swirling around this sensation were the deep, lush textures rising from the orchestra below. The amount of energy that was passing through me was incredible. I could not feel my body. It was as if I was only energy and sound. Opera it was to be then! Despite the incredible naivety with which I embarked on my chosen direction, I have been terribly lucky. I have been able to spend the last eight years working with, choreographing and directing singers in opera houses all over the world. It has been a real joy.

During this time, I have been able to work with and observe many of my contemporaries who now dance with opera companies as I had done. To be able to watch dancers from the outside, so to speak, confirmed and consolidated many of my thoughts and decisions. Early on in my new career, I was rehearsing a small group of dancers for a new opera. Occasionally, we would disappear to a quiet studio located on the sixth floor of the opera house to perfect the choreography and timing. On this particular occasion, we only had a short time to rehearse before our contribution would be seen by the management, so we were all keen to get it right. However, one dancer was missing. Time was running out and I was angry at being let down. Eventually we found her waiting in the dressing room as if nothing was wrong. When I asked her why she wasn't at rehearsal, she explained that she had a problem with her knees. I told her she should have let me know earlier. 'Oh no,' she said. 'If I'd climbed the six flights of stairs to the rehearsal room, my knees would not have made it through the perfor-

mance later. I have to pace myself.' I didn't know what to say. I could see myself in this self-deception, to dance against all odds. I felt surer than ever that my decision to be able to walk mountains in old age was the only sane path to have taken.

It was naturally not very long before I started to apply the ideas and images that I had used myself as a dancer, to help the singers and their performance. Although singing is a long way from ballet, there are many similarities in the process and the training. Singers spend an unbalanced proportion of their lives developing, listening to and worrying about their voices. They can not really hear what they are producing and so, like a dancer, become dependent on an external 'ear'. Other people's tastes, criticisms, compliments and reviews all help them piece together a sense of what works and what is appreciated, but this leaves them very insecure and full of an inner dialogue that only serves to undermine their efforts. The resulting tensions and blocks in their energy hamper their performance still further.

As I worked with the singers, I became aware of a new skill. I realized I could actually see the energy in other people's bodies. I could sense its quality and where they were constricting it, where it was blocked. I started to add images to my directing to help the singers release the energy so that it flowed throughout their entire bodies, hinting at where they were tense or where they might try to open by breathing into their body. I wanted them to sing out of every pore, as this was the only way that they were going to communicate and release their energy and their talents unbound to the audience. In some extreme instances, my own body would act as a receptor and mirror and actually appear to parallel their tension and blocked energy.

Early on in this process I was rehearsing a group of singers who were stood around me in a circle. I became aware of an incredible tightness in my chest and jaw, like a constricting band, and I could hardly breathe. Standing directly behind me was a young Welsh singer who had been both a rugby player and coal miner. Without turning around to look at him, I said: 'Richard, will you please let go of your chest and jaw. It's killing me, I can't breathe!' Everyone was pretty surprised, not least of all Richard, because when I turned around his eyes were full of tears and his lip was quivering as he told me he had never been able to let go before in his life, he had always been fighting. A couple of the female singers went spontaneously to give him a hug and tell him it was all right if he cried. Now I try to be a little less dramatic! I gently encourage the person to release the block, trying not to give away any sense of my own physical discomfort.

I was fascinated by this new skill and began to watch people's energy incessantly, not just in the theatre but also outside. I had to spend some time in Dallas, Texas, and while I was there I went along to the local YMCA to do my exercises. I found myself disturbed by the constricted energy and punishing routine of the weights room and the restrictive nature of this conventional exercise. It particularly pained me to see so many retired people being pum-

melled into shape by teenage instructors and made to do exercises that were so inappropriate to them and to their stage of life. I would stand in the corner of the gym, swinging and circling and arcing rhythmically in my own series of exercises, trying to be as unobtrusive as possible. I was viewed with suspicion by most as they all made their way through the same weights exercises, one after another.

I habitually watched one woman of about 65 who carried with her such a sense of grace and joy in her movements that her energy seemed to radiate. We struck up a conversation as she came over to tell me how beautiful she found my movements and asked if I would would show her some of them, which I gladly did. After a period back in England I returned to Dallas and to my morning routine at the gym. I looked out for my radiant friend as I exercised. When I eventually spotted her I was shocked to see that she was the shadow of her former self. Her energy was small and seemed dull, and she looked crushed and contracted as she trudged around the gym. I could not contain myself. 'What on earth has happened to you?' I blurted out. Nothing dramatic had happened in her life, but she confessed that she did not feel as free as she used to.

We sat down on the exercise mat and I gave her some exercises to open and release, to breathe and try to change the direction of the energy flow. Bless her, I saw some of the light start to return as we worked, she was so grateful. 'Now what have you been doing?' I asked her. We worked our way around the gym as she showed me the weights' exercises she had been assigned. After four or five exercises, I suddenly said, 'That's it, it's that one.' It was a pectoral pumping exercise where you pull weights forwards in front of your chest. 'I knew it,' she shouted, so excited to have confirmed that knowing voice inside her. The exercise had totally contracted and closed off the energy normally flowing across her chest, the front of her face and from the top of her head. I told her that in her 65 years she understood her body better than an 18-year-old instructress and that she must trust that knowingness. We stood back in the gym and I very wickedly described to her and got her to see the energy field of the instructress. She giggled as she saw how contracted and deformed it was from all that pumping. Superficially the body looked 'toned', but I would have described it as pinched or armour-plated.

I began to apply this new knowledge increasingly in my work in the theatre where it became known as 'Energy' work. The first time I systematically put it into practice was during a new work for Covent Garden's studio opera. The work, entitled The Dancer Hotoke, was an unforgivingly minimalist work based on a Japanese Noh opera story. The first time I listened to it, it was clear that there was very little action per se and that what it required was a 'charged' stillness from the performers. I was unsure where to begin, since many performers experience stillness as empty, without energy. If the stage were full of five singers with this concept of stillness, the piece would have been like a black hole and would simply have died on its feet. I decided that the only thing I could do was to attempt to give the singers a crash course during the four weeks of rehearsal. I would try to get them to understand energy by giving them images so that they could visualize it, develop an awareness of the energetic connection between themselves and the other performers on stage and harness and control the flow of energy in performance.

We worked for half an hour every morning, using the exercises and images now contained in the Energy Fountain chapter in this book. I was able to draw on and refer to the sensations and images that they experienced in these half-hour sessions as I directed the work. Much to my surprise, the singers responded rapidly to this approach and progressed in leaps and bounds. With a few simple images for visualizing energy, their bodies took on a sense of unity and wholeness. Whereas previously the singers had been a series of disparate parts – voice, limbs, eyes, counting, worrying – they now became compelling to watch. The images gave them an awareness of their whole self beyond the body and its role within the piece. It was as if they had been blurred and had now gelled into focus.

From the singers' point of view, they were surprised that an extra half-hour's rehearsal, which initially had seemed like an unnecessary burden, actually had the effect of increasing their energy for the whole day so that the rehearsals felt effortless. Their focus and concentration for the entire six hours of rehearsal was unfaltering. All of this was obviously very nice for us, but would anyone else notice, I wondered? The proof of the pudding was in the eating. I did not have to wait very long. The audience's reaction was wonderful. It was as if they were compelled to watch the 'charged' action, although seemingly unsure why. The Observer wrote: 'Judging by the breathless hush, I was not alone in being transfixed.' This was sufficient to convince me of the direction of my work from that point on. As if to confirm that new direction, this little obscure production was nominated for a Laurence Olivier award for outstanding achievement in opera, side by side with the lavish productions of the major houses.

Opera singers, like many people today, are concerned with being slim and fit. For some it is almost becoming an obsession as they try to fight off the traditional image of an opera singer and be taken seriously as a credible actor. Singing, though, is an athletic job and requires plenty of sustenance, physical stamina and discipline. It was not long therefore before I started to get enquiries from singers and colleagues about what kept me slim, fit, full of vitality and smiling, despite our schedules and travelling. 'Twenty minutes!' they said disbelievingly, looking at my dancer-like figure. 'Yes 20 minutes, but done every day with the right attention,' I replied.

Despite my injury and the process of healing that I had led myself through, once I was back to reasonable physical health I seemed mysteriously to forget that I contained my own answers. I continued my search for other forms of sustainable exercise, preferring to be told what to do by someone else rather than having to struc-

ture and create it for myself. It was much easier to give away my power to an existing method than to believe in my own ideas. I therefore went to a sports injury clinic, who suggested a two-hour daily workout. 'Give me 20 minutes a day,' I said, 'and I'll do it, but this two-hour workout each day is unreal. I am constantly failing, since I never achieve it. I have a life, and I can't live in the gym.' They were utterly inflexible. Two hours or nothing it seemed.

At least the clinic believed in working around injuries and had been shocked at the idea of simply taking out the bones in my feet. This inspired me with some confidence. To help my joints, they decided the best programme would be to pump up all my muscles so much that I would hardly use my joints as shock absorbers at all. That was a very strange experience, like walking everywhere wearing amazingly bouncy trainers. Very pleasant, but unsustainable. They had developed the healing of injury into a science. They measured all my muscles for 'normalcy' and I discovered I had inner thigh muscles weaker than a 'normal' woman of my height and weight, and outer thigh muscles stronger than a 'normal' man! The remedy was to hammer the weak muscles so that they caught up with the others. In hindsight, I realize how clever my body was to have compensated like that for a natural weakness.

I persisted with the programme. I was in the gym at 6.45am every day. I tried to find a joy and intention in the movements, but I have to say that even half asleep as I was at that time in the morning, I found the exercises mind-numbingly boring. They could be performed totally mechanically without engaging myself at all. I was not that long into the programme when I found I had developed a new injury – a severe hand strain from lifting weights. 'Let's take a look at it. My word, no wonder,' they said. My hands were apparently much too slender for their size and length and longer than the hands of a 'normal' man of my height. My fine hands had been one of the features of my dancing and were rather long and graceful. I did not want them pumping up to a 'normal' strength so that I could lift weights. My dawn commitment to my two-hour programme began to wain and very soon it dwindled entirely.

In response to my own needs and that of my colleagues for a gentle form of exercise that was flexible, could be done anywhere and yet be effective, I began to compile my knowledge of energy and the way that I harmonize that understanding through the daily exercises that I developed during my process of healing. I wanted to give people the tools to understand and to work intuitively with their own individual bodies. Since I have been to the extremes of athleticism and physicality and back, I wanted to share something of that process. To share the understanding that our own thoughts and imagination are the greatest tools that we have to undermine and destroy or to create and to heal our bodies. I wanted to condense the knowledge of more than 30 years of working with energy and bodies and render it accessible, practical and easy to follow for anyone who would like to be sensitively fit. The result is The Energy Source, a method of gentle daily exercise based on self-love, respect and a belief that your body carries its own wisdom. The work encourages the ability to listen to your own body, to allow it the space to heal itself and be healthy. The exercises are very flexible and can be adapted to different bodies and requirements, allowing as much or as little time commitment as is available.

To my own surprise, having used this approach consistently now for the last seven years, I am healthier and have more vitality than I ever had at the peak of my athleticism. Oh yes, and my foot injury. I have not had a peep of trouble from it since! Illness and injury can be very creative. It seems we invariably contract exactly the right complaint to make us get the message as speedily as possible. How clever the body is. I suppose the foot injury served its purpose very well.

GLOSSARY

ARCH THE BACK A backward movement of the spine that should be done with caution. Lift tall out of the waist and hips, open the chest to the ceiling and incline the upper spine, head and neck backwards slightly. This movement should feel lifted and supported in the stomach and under the shoulder blades and not sunk down or contracted in the lower back.

BREATHE THROUGH THE STIFFNESS Using the image of the outward flow of the 'out' breath to rid the body of its toxins and tension during stretching. The focus is on energy and breath flowing through the stiff area and beyond.

BRUSH THROUGH THE FLOOR In any exercise where you slowly extend one leg, push down into the floor slightly as you extend the leg and you will feel a resistance from the floor. Keep pressing into the floor as you extend the leg until only the tips of the toes remain on the floor. This is a strengthening movement. The same action should be applied in reverse as the feet come together again.

CENTRE OVER THE TOES To distribute the weight evenly over the toes. When raising onto half foot (lifting the heels), it is very easy to push the ankles either inwards or outwards, sending the weight of the body out over the little toes or inwards over the big toe joint. Try to rise up in a direct straight line through the arches of the feet, keeping the ankles strong, so that the weight of the body is evenly distributed over all the toes.

CENTRE THE WEIGHT To distribute the weight evenly over the feet. In the standing position, it is a common mistake to carry the weight forwards over the toes or backwards into the heels. Either of these creates a distortion in the posture and spine and affects our readiness for movement. Before starting an exercise, rock your weight slightly forwards on the feet then slightly backwards and then back to centre, until you are aware that your weight is evenly distributed over the whole foot.

CURL THE PELVIS A rolling movement of the pelvis and hips which affects the position of the spine. If you move the pelvis forwards and up, the lower back will curve. If you move it backwards and up, then the lower back will arch. The Energy Source exercises use only the forward roll of the pelvis in order to stretch or protect the lower back in certain movements. This movement feels like a curling up or a tucking under of the sitting bones as the spine curves.

CURVE THE BACK To gently bend forwards, starting by lowering the head and neck, then releasing the shoulders and following with the spine, so that it bends forwards one vertebra at a time.

DIAGONAL An imaginary line that is at a 45-degree angle to the body. If you are facing a wall, to reach out to the diagonals would be to reach to the left and right corners of the room.

ENERGY BLOCK An area in the body that is either habitually held in a state of tension or is temporarily tense and contracted. An energy block results in the area being 'cut off' from the rest of the body and from the free flow of energy. If left unattended, this can manifest itself as permanent postural change, general loss of energy and wellbeing or illness in that area.

ENERGY FIELD An area of energy directly surrounding the physical body that you impact as you move and breathe. The size and quality of the energy field is personal to the individual and changeable according to emotions and circumstances. It can normally be sensed as an oval around the body, extending two to four feet (60–120cm) away from the surface.

FACE FRONT To stand with your feet, hips, shoulders and head all facing the same direction. Choose a direction that you will refer to as 'front' when you start an exercise and always begin from and return to this direction.

FEET PARALLEL To stand with your toes pointing directly out in front of you so that they are in line with the knees and hips.

FIVE POINTS This refers to the points of the body through which you consciously draw or send energy, from or into your energy field. The points are the feet, the hands and the crown of the head.

FLEX THE FOOT To tilt the foot and toes up towards the shin, sending energy out through the back of the leg and the ball of the heel.

FORWARD OF THE BODY LINE This term is used to describe the position of the arms in certain exercises. Imagine the side view of your body is a vertical line. Lift the arms to the sides and hold them slightly forwards of that line so that you are just aware of them out of the corners of your eyes.

HIPS SQUARE/STRAIGHT This is when both hip bones are level and pointing to the front. In many exercises you are asked to keep the hips square, despite other spiralling or twisting movements in the upper body.

'IN' BREATH/'OUT' BREATH The exercises consciously combine the breath with the movements. To exercise effectively you need to maintain an awareness of the breathing and a control of the rhythm of the breathing. The 'out' breath is the most important for the Energy Source work, to empty the lungs completely, helping rid the body of toxins and tension. The filling of the lungs, the 'in' breath, is a natural reflex action. The breathing acts as a facilitator for the movement of energy in the body. The freer and stronger the breathing, the clearer the flow of energy through and beyond the body.

INFLATE THE SPINE/LEGS On a long 'in' breath, imagine that you are drawing the air up through your body from the earth. The air lifts and straightens the legs from out of a bend or uncurls the spine as it inflates and lifts one vertebra after another.

KEEP THE FEET SOFT A common tendency is to grip the floor with the toes, contracting and tightening the tendons and muscles of the feet and ankles. This prevents a clear flow of energy into the body from the earth and is a brittle stance that can lead to injury. To keep the feet soft means to consciously release them and to let them open and spread across the floor.

KEEP THE MOVEMENT FLUID To keep an image of an outward flow of water or light energy through the limbs while moving or exercising. This prevents the muscles going rigid with the effort and so blocking the energy flow.

LIFT OUT OF THE HIPS/WAIST To consciously carry the weight of the upper body so that the waist and hips are elongated, enabling the lower body to move more freely.

LISTENING IN To stand still for an instant and to focus on the physical sensations within the body and on the rhythm and quality of the breathing.

LOCKED This most commonly refers to the knees or the elbows, but could be applied to any joint. A joint may be locked if it is overextended, for instance if you over-straighten the arms or legs. The limb and joint reach a position that feels secure, but which is in fact brittle and immobile. Exercises done with locked joints can cause injury, so take care to release the joint a little and send energy out through the limb so that the limb feels strong but fluid.

MIND'S EYE The part of the mind or imagination that can create and retain an image. Also a consciousness that can be focused inwards and perceive bodily sensations.

OPEN THE CHEST TO THE CEILING As you breathe in, expand and soften the front of the chest, then tilt the breastbone slightly upwards towards the ceiling. Let the upper body arch a little, tilting the head back as a natural extention of the spine. Hold the arms up to form a circle in front, palms facing the chest, to balance the backward movement of the upper body.

OPEN STAR STANDING The finishing position of The Star preparatory exercise, where you stand with the chest and sholders wide and arms raised and reaching out to both sides. This is one of the most open positions for the body, which allows energy to flow freely through the body, passing in and out through the five points of The Star.

POINT OF FOCUS An object or point of visual reference at eye level in front of you on which you can concentrate while exercising. The point of focus helps to balance and stabilize the movement and concentrates the energy and intention of the exercise.

RAISE ONTO HALF FOOT To raise the heels as high as is comfortable, so that the weight of the body is shifted onto the toes. Make sure your weight is evenly distributed over the toes. This movement is normally done with an 'out' breath, sending the breath and energy down through the legs and out through the feet into the earth like strong roots.

REACH TO THE CORNERS Assuming that you are directly facing a wall, to reach out to the corners is to reach out with the limbs or upper body at a 45-degree angle to the body, as if reaching towards the corners of the room. This is otherwise known as the diagonal.

RESIST THE LOWERING/ BENDING/ STRAIGHTENING This means to work against yourself or against gravity by consciously resisting the movement. If applied consistently, this helps strengthen and lengthen the muscles. For example, to resist the lowering of the heels from half foot means to consciously lift up and lengthen the body as the heels slowly lower to the floor and not to succumb to gravity and experience the lowering as a collapse.

RETURN TO CENTRE In this programme, centre refers to an upright, vertical posture with the body facing front. If standing, your weight should be evenly distributed on both feet. So, after curving the spine or stretching to the side, you would return to centre.

Glossary

SHAKE OUT To vibrate and loosen the muscles of a limb that has been working intensely, or to deliberately shake tension and blocked energy out of the body back into the earth.

SUPPORTING LEG In exercises that work one leg at a time, the supporting leg refers to the leg that you stand on. This takes the whole weight of the body, leaving the other leg free. Check that the supporting knee is not locked and rigid, that the supporting foot is soft and alive throughout and that your weight is lifted up out of your hips and supporting leg and not sunk down onto them.

SWING A movement that begins in the centre of the body, where the limbs and/or upper body follow naturally, using the momentum of their relaxed weight.

TURN THE FEET OUT A standing position where the heels remain touching but the feet separate a little so that the toes are pointing outwards to the diagonals. In this position the backs of the legs should also be touching.

UNCURL TO STANDING To raise the spine up from a curved forwards position. The movement starts at the base of the spine. Using one long, drawn out 'in' breath, imagine filling the spine with the breath and lifting it one vertebra at a time. The neck and the head are the last to unfold to upright.

WORKING LEG In exercises that work with one leg at a time, this refers to the leg that is isolated and exercising. These exercises alternate sides so that each leg can be isolated and worked in turn.

THE ENERGY SOURCE RETREAT
Costa Blanca, Spain

Easter and Summer holidays and courses in unspoilt Javea.
For information write to:

Clare West
The Energy Source Retreat
Box No. 374
Ctra. Cabo La Nao (PLA) 71-6
03730 Javea,
Alicante, Spain

Or telephone UK 01273 723130

Energy Programme Notes

Energy Programme Notes

Energy Programme Notes

Energy Programme Notes

Energy Programme Notes

Energy Programme Notes

Energy Programme Notes